A NEW NORMAL

A T1D Mom Shares
Facts, Tips, & Advice
About
Type 1 Diabetes

Laurie Pearlman Park

DISCLAIMER

The information in this book is intended to help readers gain a general understanding of Type 1 diabetes.

Type 1 diabetes treatment is highly personalized. For diagnosis and treatment of Type 1 diabetes or any other medical illness or condition, consult your own physician. This book is not intended to be a substitute for treatment by, or the advice and care of, your own physician.

The information, advice, and tips contained in this book are based upon the research and personal experiences of the author. While the author has tried to ensure that the information presented is accurate and up to date, she shall not be held responsible for any loss, damage, or adverse effects of any kind resulting from reliance on the contents herein.

NOTES ON WRITING STYLE

The author intentionally avoided referring to a person with Type 1 diabetes as a "Type 1 diabetic" to be sensitive to some people who feel that the term labels and defines someone by their illness, when they are, of course, much more than just their illness.

In order to avoid repetition, "Type 1 diabetes" is referred to in this book by that term or by "T1D," "Type 1," and occasionally, simply as "diabetes." Similarly, "a person with Type 1 diabetes" is referred to by that term or as a "person with T1D," a "person with Type 1," or simply, a "PWD" (person with diabetes).

To acknowledge both male and female genders, the author chose to alternate between the use of male and female pronouns according to chapter.

Words in boldface and italic are defined in the Glossary beginning on page 101.

for Jenny, of course

Contents

Preface

"*I don't have time for the nervous breakdown I deserve.*"

When my daughter, Jenny, was diagnosed with Type 1 diabetes (T1D), I felt like both of us had been hit by a truck. You probably did too. Type 1 diabetes wasn't anywhere on my radar screen. There was no history of it on either side of the family. The diagnosis explained her ravenous appetite and irritability in the previous months, but that was little consolation when I started to learn how difficult Type 1 management was. She was going to need insulin injections, multiple times a day, every day, for the rest of her life -- just to stay alive!

After three days in the hospital, she was discharged and my husband and I became responsible for her daily diabetes care. Inconceivably, the medical professionals expected us to test her blood sugar, give her insulin injections, record the type and quantity of food she ate, the activity she did, and her blood sugar levels in response to that food or activity, determine the right amount of insulin she would need for each meal and snack, wake up twice in the middle of the night to check her blood sugar, and more -- on top of our existing jobs, responsibilities, and lives in general. There was simply no time to let the diagnosis sink in or gradually adjust to our family's "new normal."

A few weeks after the diagnosis, I saw a meme which said: "I don't have time for the nervous breakdown I deserve." I chuckled sadly to myself because that was exactly how I felt. I *didn't* have time for the nervous breakdown I deserved … because I was scrambling every hour of the day just to keep my child alive!

As devastated as I was, there was also no question in my mind that I was going to do everything in my power to manage her Type 1 correctly, protect her from complications, and enable her to lead a "normal," happy, healthy, and long life.

I read the leading books, blogs, and websites about Type 1 diabetes. I searched the Internet for information and promising research. I made mistakes and learned from them. I got to know other Type 1 parents, many of whom were further along in their journeys than I was. Their strength, support, and success stories inspired me.

The more I learned, the more optimistic and in control I felt. I discovered that some of my worst fears about T1D were unfounded and were based on outdated information. Scientists had made great advances with the medicines, devices, and technologies used to treat Type 1 diabetes, and treatment was continuing to improve quickly. Long-term medical problems as a result of having T1D were no longer inevitable. Many people who had T1D for decades had *no* complications from the disease. People with Type 1 diabetes were healthy and thriving -- physically, intellectually, and emotionally. They had careers and personal lives just like everyone else. Not only was knowledge key to managing Type 1 successfully, but it was also key to coping with the emotional aspects of having a child with T1D.

When Jenny was diagnosed, I felt like life would never be good again, but I was wrong! Of course, having T1D is hard, but we were never going to just wave a white flag and surrender. We learned and we adjusted. We sought help and support. We emerged from a dark place, feeling stronger and hopeful, to **A New Normal**. You can too.

Chapter 1

What is Type 1 Diabetes?

> *"Nah, not doing it." - my pancreas*
>
> *"Yes, I have Type 1 diabetes.*
> *No, it is not because I ate too much sugar."*
>
> *News flash: T1D and T2D are not the same!*

1. *Type 1 diabetes (T1D)* is a disease in which the *pancreas* stops making *insulin,* a hormone which regulates *blood sugar* levels.[1]

2. People need insulin to live. Since people with Type 1 diabetes don't make their own insulin, they must get their insulin from an external source. To do this, they must *inject* insulin or *pump* insulin through a medical device into their bodies every single day.

3. Type 1 diabetes used to be called "juvenile diabetes," but "Type 1 diabetes" is now the preferred name. "Juvenile" was eliminated to reflect the fact that the disease can strike children or adults at any age, although it more commonly strikes in childhood, adolescence, or young adulthood.

---

[1] Sometimes, after a T1D diagnosis has been made and insulin injections have begun, the pancreas will start to produce some of its own insulin again for a limited period of time. This is called the "***honeymoon phase,***" and a patient whose pancreas is producing some insulin is said to be "honeymooning."

4. **T1D is treated with insulin. Insulin is not a cure for T1D; it is a treatment which allows the disease to be managed.**

5. **Type 1 diabetes is a *chronic* illness, meaning that it is lifelong and will never "go away."** It is not an illness which patients will outgrow.

6. **Type 1 is an *autoimmune* disease, that is, it occurs because the patient's own immune system mistakenly attacks and destroys the insulin-producing *beta cells* in the patient's own pancreas.**

7. **No one knows exactly what causes T1D, but scientists believe that both genetic and environmental factors are involved.** More specifically, there is a genetic predisposition for a person to develop Type 1 and an environmental trigger which makes it happen.

8. **Type 1 diabetes is not anyone's fault. T1D is NOT caused by eating too much sugar, being overweight, not exercising enough, or anything else related to diet or lifestyle.**

9. **Type 1 cannot be prevented or reversed.**

10. **T1D is not contagious.**

11. **Type 1 diabetes accounts for approximately 5% of all diabetes cases. *Type 2 diabetes (T2D)* is much more common and accounts for approximately 95% of all diabetes cases.** (In addition to Type 1 and Type 2, there are also several other types of diabetes which are not covered in this book.)

12. **Often, people mistakenly equate Type 1 diabetes with Type 2 diabetes, but in fact, they are not the same.** They have different causes and different treatments. People with Type 1 diabetes have stopped making their own insulin, so all people with Type 1 must inject or pump insulin. People with Type 2 still make their own insulin, but have become resistant to it and do not use it efficiently; most people with Type 2 do *not* have to inject or pump insulin.

13. **Nearly 1.6 million Americans have T1D, according to a 2020 report by the Centers for Disease Control (CDC). That represents a nearly 30% increase in T1D diagnoses since 2017.**

The CDC previously reported that between 2001 and 2009, there was a 21% increase in the prevalence of T1D in people under age 20. The reason for these increases is unknown.

14. Living with Type 1 diabetes is challenging and requires a lot of work, but millions of people do it successfully. Advances in treatments and technologies mean that today, people can live active, full, productive, healthy, and long lives with T1D. There is virtually no limit to one's achievement despite the illness.

T1D mom tip: Type 1 diabetes is not the same as Type 2 diabetes. Most people don't understand that. When someone says something about T1D which is factually wrong, I use it as an opportunity to educate them and to raise awareness about T1D.

Summary

- Type One diabetes is an illness in which the body has stopped making insulin.
- People with T1D must inject or pump insulin into their bodies every single day for the rest of their lives.
- Type 1 is an autoimmune illness. It is not contagious.
- T1D isn't related to diet, exercise, or lifestyle, and isn't anyone's fault.
- Type 1 diabetes and Type 2 diabetes are very different illnesses.
- With proper **management**, people with T1D can live lives like everyone else.

Chapter 2

Signs and Symptoms of Type 1 Diabetes; Diabetic Ketoacidosis (DKA)

> *Step 1. Drink*
> *Step 2: Pee*
> *Step 3: Repeat Steps 1 and 2*

1. The first signs and symptoms of Type 1 diabetes usually develop quickly, over a period of weeks. They are:

- **extreme thirst;**
- **frequent urination (sometimes seen in babies and young children as a heavy diaper or bedwetting);**
- **increased appetite/ constant hunger;**
- **unexplained weight loss;**
- **blurry vision[2]**
- **fatigue/ tiredness; and**
- **irritability/ mood changes**

2. If not correctly diagnosed and treated, Type 1 diabetes can progress to *diabetic ketoacidosis (DKA)*, a very serious, life-threatening condition. DKA can occur when a person with T1D doesn't have enough insulin in her system. *Glucose* builds up in the bloodstream, and the body reacts by using its own fat for fuel, turning it into harmful substances called *ketones*. When ketones accumulate in the bloodstream at high levels, a patient can go into DKA.

---

[2] Blurry vision from undiagnosed T1D is a temporary problem and will resolve on its own after a few weeks or months of insulin therapy.

Symptoms of DKA include those listed above, plus:

- **stomach/ abdominal pain;**
- **nausea and vomiting;**
- **fruity odor on breath; and**
- **rapid, heavy breathing**

3. Diabetic ketoacidosis is a medical emergency which requires immediate treatment in a hospital. Left untreated, DKA can lead to organ failure and be fatal within hours or days. Approximately one-third of children with T1D are already in DKA when they are diagnosed with Type 1 diabetes.

4. People with T1D who run very high blood sugars are at risk of DKA at any time, not just at the time of diagnosis.

5. People in DKA usually have both ketones and high blood sugar levels. It is possible, however, for a person with Type 1 who has ketones to be in DKA even if her blood sugar level isn't very high at the time she is tested.

6. It's common for parents to feel guilty if they missed or misinterpreted signs of undiagnosed T1D in their children. If that is the way you feel, try not to beat yourself up over it. (There have been cases in which trained health care providers have mistaken T1D symptoms for a stomach bug, strep throat, a growth spurt, or a urinary tract infection.) Remember: T1D is not anyone's fault. Don't waste your energy feeling guilty; instead, try to channel it into learning about T1D and how to manage it.

<u>T1D mom confession</u>: When our family was on vacation at the beach last summer, I scolded my daughter for drinking all the water in the thermos I brought for the entire family to share. Little did I know that it was undiagnosed T1D which was causing her extreme thirst.

<u>T1D dad confession</u>: Before diagnosis, I knew that something wasn't quite right with my son. He was irritable and moody. We had just moved to a new state and he had started a new school, so I chalked it up to the stress of the move. It never occurred to me that he might have had T1D.

<u>T1D mom confession</u>: My six-year-old had been potty-trained since he was three, then out of nowhere, he started wetting the bed every night. I had no idea that it was because he had T1D.

<u>T1D dad confession</u>: My wife and I initially thought that our teenage daughter's constant hunger was due to an eating disorder. A few months later, we learned that it was a symptom of T1D.

<u>Summary</u>

- Symptoms of T1D include excessive thirst, frequent urination, tiredness, and weight loss.
- Undiagnosed T1D can progress to diabetic ketoacidosis, a life-threatening condition which requires immediate medical treatment.

Chapter 3

Initial Diagnosis and Hospital Stay

> *"Zombies ate my son's pancreas and the diabetes team expects me to give him seven shots a day?*
> *I must be dreaming."*

1. A Type 1 diabetes diagnosis is made based on lab tests showing high *blood glucose* (*BG*, aka blood sugar), the presence of ketones, and an elevated *A1c* test result. A1c is a blood test which measures a person's average overall *blood glucose level* for the previous 2 - 3 months.

2. Once T1D is diagnosed, it is treated immediately with insulin. The patient may initially be given insulin intravenously to quickly reduce blood sugar levels and ketones.

3. In the United States, newly-diagnosed patients are usually admitted to the hospital, where they will stay for a few days to get treatment and to learn about Type 1 diabetes.

4. Soon after diagnosis, patients (if old enough to understand) and parents/ caregivers begin their initial diabetes education with a crash course about Type 1 diabetes and its management. Don't feel embarrassed to ask questions or admit that you do not understand something. A patient or parent of a child with T1D must understand and be able to perform basic diabetes management before leaving the hospital. (Additional T1D education and training will take place in the coming weeks and months.)

5. When a child with Type 1 is discharged from the hospital, the parents are responsible for managing the child's diabetes. In very young children, parents must do all the diabetes management. Depending on the child's age and ability, he may be able to participate *to some degree* in his own diabetes management. Ultimately, though, it is the parents' responsibility to make sure that their minor child's T1D is being managed correctly.

By no means are parents expected to be perfect at managing their child's diabetes. Nearly all parents will make mistakes, especially in the beginning, and they will learn from them.

If, however, it becomes apparent that a parent is not managing or overseeing his child's diabetes care, and the child's health is seriously endangered, then there are grounds for authorities to investigate and to take action to protect the child.

T1D mom confession: Initially, I was shocked that my son had Type 1 diabetes. No one in our family had it, and I really didn't even know what Type 1 was. When the diabetes educator taught us about T1D and showed me how I was going to have to test my son's blood sugar and give him multiple shots every single day, my brain simply couldn't process the information. Thank goodness that my husband was there and was able to understand it all.

Summary

- Once a person's Type 1 diabetes diagnosis is confirmed, insulin treatment begins.
- Patients and their parents are given a "crash course" on Type 1.
- A person with T1D or parent of a child with T1D should be able to perform basic diabetes management before the patient is discharged from the hospital.

Chapter 4

Leaving the Hospital and Going Home

> *"I went to bed at 10 pm and slept deeply throughout the night," said no T1D parent ever.*

1. After a few days in the hospital for treatment and education, the patient will go home.

2. **You will probably leave the hospital with some diabetes supplies, written information including instructions about T1D management, and other materials like log sheets to record blood sugar levels and insulin doses. You should have a clear understanding of what you are expected to do in the next few days.**

3. **Make sure that you have the telephone number to reach the diabetes team in non-emergency and emergency situations, and that you understand when and why you should call a member of the team. Most parents of children with T1D are instructed to call a diabetes team member every day for the first few weeks to report blood sugar levels.**

4. **Stop at a pharmacy on the way home to fill all of the diabetes prescriptions the patient has been given.**

5. **Buy a food scale.** A basic food scale which measures in both *grams* (metric system) and ounces is adequate. It costs about $10 and is sold in stores like Target, Wal-Mart, and Bed Bath & Beyond. If your budget allows, you may want to pay more for a food scale with additional features such as pre-programmed nutrition information. If you don't have a measuring cup and measuring spoon, buy those too. **Weighing and measuring food are important tools in T1D management.**

6. It's common for parents to worry whether they're capable of managing their child's diabetes on their own once they are back home. They fear that they will accidentally make a mistake which will harm the child. Some say that leaving the hospital with their newly-diagnosed child feels more frightening than it felt to leave the hospital with their first newborn. Within a short time, though, parents and patients will become more competent and confident.

7. At least initially, parents will have to check their child's blood sugar overnight.

8. In the United States, the ***Family and Medical Leave Act (FMLA)*** requires government employers and most private employers with over 50 employees to give employees up to 12 weeks of unpaid time off from work ("leave") each year to care for a spouse, child, or parent with T1D. Leave under the FMLA doesn't have to be taken all at once; it can be taken intermittently for T1D doctors' appointments, required classes/ training on T1D management, and for T1D-related illness, as long as, cumulatively, the leave doesn't exceed 12 weeks per year.

Many parents who can afford to take unpaid leave find that it is particularly helpful to take some leave right after diagnosis, when diabetes management is still very new to everyone in the family.

<u>T1D mom confession</u>: When my daughter was diagnosed, I stayed in her hospital room the entire time she was there. When she was discharged, I was very scared about how I was going to be able to manage her diabetes back home on my own. I thought, "I can't believe that the medical professionals are handing this huge responsibility over to me."

<u>T1D dad tip</u>: I knew of another father in our neighborhood whose son had been diagnosed with T1D a few years before my son was diagnosed. I asked both of them to come to our house the first time we had to inject insulin on our own. Since they had years of experience, it was reassuring to have them there, confirming that we were doing everything correctly.

Summary

- It's very common for parents to feel scared when their newly-diagnosed child is discharged from the hospital.
- The day you are discharged from the hospital, fill all of your diabetes prescriptions at the pharmacy and get a food scale, a measuring cup and a measuring spoon.
- If you don't understand any aspect of diabetes management, say so. The healthcare professionals who train you understand that you have been given a lot of information in a short period of time and that the entire experience is overwhelming for most people.

Chapter 5

Insulin

Laughter is the best medicine ... unless you have Type 1 diabetes. Then insulin is definitely better.

1. Insulin is a hormone which regulates blood sugar levels. Because people with T1D have stopped making their own insulin, they need to inject or pump man-made insulin into their bodies.

2. Insulin is a treatment for diabetes. Insulin is NOT a cure; it will not make Type 1 diabetes "go away."

3. In 1921, insulin was discovered in Canada by Dr. Frederick Banting and his team of researchers. The first version of insulin which was successfully used on patients with T1D was derived from animals and purified to make it safe to be injected in human beings. Before then, Type 1 diabetes was always fatal. Each of the men who discovered insulin sold his patent rights to the University of Toronto for one dollar! Banting is reported to have explained the nominal sale price by saying, "Insulin does not belong to me, it belongs to the world."

4. There is a lot of false information on the Internet and elsewhere about "miracle cures" for T1D (cinnamon, cucumber water, okra, apple cider vinegar, special foods, gluten-free diets, exercise, etc.), or about people who had Type 1, but were cured and no longer have it. **The truth is that there is currently no cure for Type 1 diabetes. Nor has anyone who has ever had Type 1 diabetes been cured of it.**

5. The insulin formulations which most people with T1D in the United States and other developed countries use today are man-made and manufactured by drug companies. Today's insulins work far better than earlier versions of insulin used by PWD, but still do not work as well as the natural insulin made by a healthy person's pancreas.

6. Currently, insulin must be injected or *infused* with an *insulin pump* (a *pump*). Insulin can't be taken by mouth because stomach acids would destroy it before it ever reached the bloodstream. (In 2014, the FDA approved an inhalable powder insulin called Afrezza for use in adults under limited circumstances (see Chapter 27).)

7. Pancreas transplant surgery is not a routine treatment for Type 1 diabetes because it carries much greater risks -- including the risk of infection -- than the standard treatment of injecting or infusing insulin. In addition, pancreas transplant patients must take anti-rejection medication indefinitely, and the side effects of anti-rejection medication are worse than the side effects of insulin.

8. The food which we eat is broken down by the body into glucose. This glucose then enters the bloodstream. Insulin's job is to move glucose from the bloodstream into the body's cells. This is how the cells get energy to function properly.

9. The pancreas of a person who *doesn't* have Type 1 diabetes automatically senses how much glucose is in the bloodstream and produces just the right amount of insulin to move that glucose into the body's cells. The cells get the energy they need and the bloodstream no longer has too much glucose in it. This process, shown in the following diagram, is known as a ***closed loop system.***

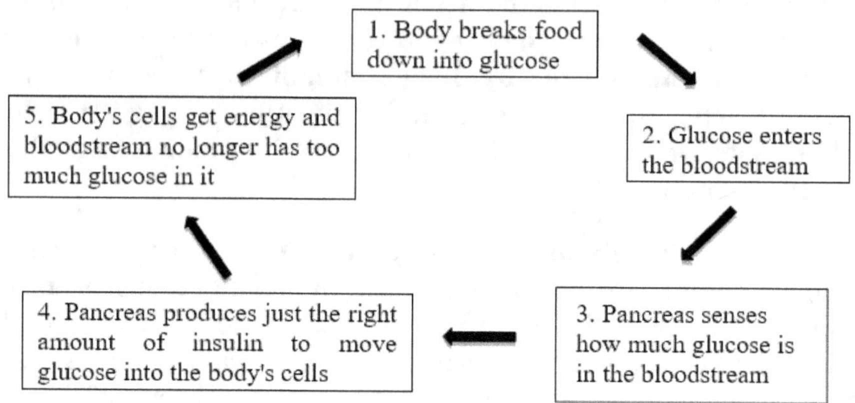

10. The body of a person with T1D doesn't automatically carry out every step in the closed loop model. The goal of the *artificial pancreas* (see Chapter 26) is to create a technology for people with Type 1 diabetes which mimics the closed loop system.

11. If a person with T1D doesn't inject or pump insulin into his body, glucose can't enter his cells. Instead, it builds up in his bloodstream. This leads to *hyperglycemia* (high blood sugar) -- too much sugar in the blood. In the short term, he will have symptoms of hyperglycemia, which may then progress to DKA. In the long term, hyperglycemia can cause serious damage to the body's small blood vessels, capillaries, and organs.

12. It is recommended that you keep unopened insulin vials and *insulin pens* in the refrigerator (between 36°F and 46°F).

13. Once you open an insulin vial or pen, you should keep it at room temperature (between 56°F and 80°F) and use it for a maximum of 28 consecutive days. Insulin manufacturers instruct users to throw out opened insulin after 28 days because it may not be effective anymore.

14. Every vial of insulin or insulin pen has an expiration date printed on it. Don't use insulin, even if it has never been opened, after its expiration date because it may not be effective anymore.

15. Know how much insulin you have left. Don't wait until you are out of insulin to request a refill.

16. A person with T1D needs insulin every single day! NEVER ration or discontinue insulin -- not even for one day! People with T1D who have rationed or stopped taking insulin have gone into DKA and some have even died.

T1D mom tip: Unopened insulin is supposed to be refrigerated. I reserve the butter compartment of our refrigerator for my son's insulin. It stays safe and doesn't get lost among other foods in the refrigerator.

T1D dad tip: Once, I accidentally dropped my son's glass insulin vial on the tile floor. The vial shattered and all the insulin spilled out. When I told another T1D dad what had happened, he told me that he wraps several wide rubber bands around his son's insulin vials to cushion and protect them if they fall.

T1D mom tip: Another T1D mom told me about insulin cooling cases, sold at many pharmacies and online. They keep insulin vials and pens in the correct temperature range. They are great to use in extreme heat or cold, or when we travel.

T1D teen tip: I went in a hot tub about half an hour after I gave myself insulin with lunch. I felt my blood sugar dropping, and quickly got out of the hot tub to confirm and treat the low. I later learned that people with Type 1 should avoid hot tubs and even very hot showers or baths because extreme heat affects the absorption rate of insulin and can lead to a low blood sugar.

Summary

- People with T1D need to inject or infuse insulin every single day.
- Always keep insulin in the recommended temperature range.
- Never use expired insulin.
- Know how much insulin you have left and don't wait until you are out of insulin to request a refill.
- NEVER ration or stop taking insulin!

Chapter 6

The Diabetes Team

When your endocrinologist asks you why
your blood sugar was high for four hours
on a Thursday evening two weeks ago...

1. A person with Type 1 diabetes will usually be treated by a multidisciplinary group of medical professionals, each with a specific role. Together, they form your diabetes team. These professionals are:

    a. ***Endocrinologist (endo)*** - a doctor who specializes in treating Type 1 diabetes. A *pediatric* endocrinologist specializes in treating children with T1D. Board-certified endocrinologists have years of advanced training to treat Type 1 and are knowledgeable about the latest advances in treatment. Some people with Type 1 diabetes go only to their ***primary care provider (PCP)*** for their T1D care. Although going to a primary care provider for T1D is better than not going to any doctor at all, it is recommended that people with T1D go to endocrinologists for their diabetes care.

    b. ***Certified Diabetes Educator (CDE)*** - a healthcare professional (usually also a nurse or dietitian) who is certified to teach PWD how to manage the disease

c. ***Dietitian (aka registered dietitian or RD)*** - a healthcare professional who teaches PWD about nutrition, how to count carbs, how to match insulin to food and drink consumed, and how to maintain, lose, or gain weight, if needed. A dietitian can help a patient plan a healthy diet which takes into account her lifestyle and personal preferences.

d. ***Ophthalmologist*** - a doctor who specializes in treating the eyes. Once every year, a person with T1D should go to an ophthalmologist to have her eyes examined for possible damage from diabetes.

e. ***Mental Health Professional*** - a professional counselor, social worker, psychologist, or psychiatrist who can help people with T1D, and their parents or caregivers, deal with the emotional aspects of Type 1 (see Preface and Chapter 32)

2. In addition to getting treatment from the diabetes team, a PWD should:

a. continue to see her PCP (pediatrician, internist, family medicine doctor, physician assistant, or nurse practitioner) for non-T1D treatment and preventive care, including getting an annual flu shot and staying up to date on other recommended immunizations; and

b. go to a dentist for a checkup and cleaning every six months (People with Type 1 are at greater risk for gum disease than people who don't have it.)

3. A person with Type 1 or her caregiver will have frequent contact with her pharmacist, who can provide information about prescription and over-the-counter medication side effects and interactions. A pharmacist can also contact your doctor and insurance company to help you get your medication if you run into problems.

4. Currently, patients with T1D are supposed to have a "diabetes checkup" once every three months, even if diabetes management is going well. Lab tests, including the A1c test, will be performed. The endocrinologist will analyze the patient's recent blood glucose readings and make any necessary changes to her diabetes management instructions.

5. The endocrinology appointment is also an opportunity to ask questions, get advice, share concerns (including any about cost and insurance issues), and request prescription refills.

6. A good endocrinologist treats her patients and their caregivers with respect. A good endocrinologist is supportive, recognizes that diabetes management is difficult, and does not shame or embarrass patients or their parents. Since a patient with Type 1 will see her endocrinologist four times a year, it's important to have a good professional relationship with the endocrinologist.

7. The patient/ endocrinologist relationship is a two-way street. The patient and her caregiver should arrive on time for appointments, follow the endocrinologist's office rules, and be polite and respectful to the endocrinologist, other members of the diabetes team, and their assistants.

T1D dad tip: We live in a rural area without any endocrinologists nearby. Even though I could take my son to his pediatrician for his Type 1 diabetes checkups, I choose to drive two hours each way so that he can see a pediatric endocrinologist at a children's hospital. I know that he gets the best possible care there.

T1D mom tip: If any member of my daughter's diabetes team is unsupportive or unreasonably critical, I will ask to see someone else at future appointments. T1D is hard to manage and my daughter will do better with someone who she feels is "on her side."

T1D teen tip: Once a year, I go to an ophthalmologist for a dilated eye exam to check for eye problems. At my most recent appointment, the ophthalmologist told me that although vision loss from Type 1 diabetes was very common in the past, today, PWD who manage their diabetes correctly should not expect to have vision loss from T1D.

T1D dad tip: Last summer, I picked up my son's insulin pens from the pharmacy and forgot to take them into the house when I got home. They sat in the summer heat in the car until the next day. I was sure that the temperature was above 90 degrees and that the insulin was no longer safe to use. I brought them back to the pharmacy and explained to the pharmacist what had happened. She had me return them to her and gave me a replacement, free of charge.

<u>Summary</u>

- A person with Type 1 diabetes should see her endocrinologist once every three months for a routine diabetes checkup.
- Nowadays, people with T1D are treated by a team of health care professionals. In addition to seeing an endocrinologist, they may see or speak with other members of the diabetes team at and between appointments.
- A person with Type 1 should have her eyes examined by an ophthalmologist once a year.
- A PWD should continue to see her primary care doctor for non-T1D matters, routine checkups and preventive care.

Chapter 7

Diabetes Management

*It's my first day on the job and I'm already
considered part of management.*

1. Taking care of your (or your child's) Type 1 diabetes is called "managing diabetes." **Managing T1D minimizes the effects of the disease.**

2. Proper diabetes management consists of:

    a. frequent blood sugar testing;
    b. injecting or infusing insulin;
    c. paying attention to the quantity of ***carbohydrate*** consumed; and
    d. treating high and low blood sugars (highs and lows)

3. The man-made insulins which PWD use today are better than older formulations, but are not as good as the insulin which a healthy pancreas produces naturally.

It is therefore unrealistic to expect a PWD to be able to keep his blood sugar in his ***target range*** -- the desired range of blood sugar levels specified by one's endocrinologist -- *at all times*. Instead, the goal is to keep blood sugar in the target range *most of the time*, without having too many high or low blood sugars.

4. Diabetes management today is very different than it was in the past. Up until the early 1990s, most doctors instructed patients with T1D to give themselves only one or two insulin shots a day.

a. In 1993, a major clinical trial called the *Diabetes Control and Complications Trial (DCCT)* changed the way Type 1 diabetes was treated.

b. The DCCT compared two groups of patients:

(1) the **Standard Management** group, which followed the standard treatment *at that time* (only one or two insulin injections a day); and

(2) the ***Intensive Management*** group, which tested their blood sugar more often, injected or infused insulin more often, followed a diet and exercise plan, adjusted insulin doses according to the food they ate and the exercise they did, and had more frequent checkups with a multi-disciplinary diabetes team

c. **The DCCT proved that Intensive Management was much better than Standard Management.** After ten years, people in the Intensive Management group had:

(1) lower A1c's;
(2) a dramatically lower rate of long-term *complications* from diabetes; and
(3) slower progression of any existing complications

5. Intensive management (aka *intensive treatment*) leads to what is called *tight control.* Intensive management requires PWD to spend **MORE** time and do **MORE** work managing their diabetes than patients had to do before the DCCT. The DCCT, however, proved that spending extra time and effort on diabetes management is worth it because it dramatically reduces the risk of long-term complications from T1D.

Today, many people with Type 1 diabetes who have practiced intensive management and have had tight control have no diabetes complications at all!

T1D dad tip: There will be times when I manage my daughter's diabetes exactly as I should, but she will still have a high or a low blood sugar. I used to get discouraged when this happened, but now I realize that Type 1 can be unpredictable and I won't get it right every single time.

T1D mom tip: Successful diabetes management means making sure that my son always has all his diabetes supplies on him or nearby.

T1D dad tip: If, like me, you wondered why it was necessary for your child to have to get SEVEN insulin shots a day, the answer is that doing so will greatly reduce his risk of long-term complications, i.e., it will keep him much healthier for a longer period of time. Although there is no ironclad guarantee, our children may never have any long-term complications from diabetes.

Summary

- Putting in the recommended time and effort of intensive diabetes management dramatically reduces long-term complications from Type 1 diabetes.
- Today, many people with T1D who practice intensive management and have tight control have no diabetes complications at all.

Chapter 8

Hyperglycemia and
What Raises Blood Sugar

"I love the expressions on people's faces when we are out in public and my mother casually asks me if I'm high!"

Blood sugar -- the abbreviation is B.S. for a reason!

1. Hyperglycemia means high blood sugar -- too much glucose (sugar) in the blood. A patient doesn't feel well when her blood sugar is too high. Very high blood sugar can progress to a life-threatening condition called diabetic ketoacidosis (DKA). In the long term, very high blood sugar can also lead to serious medical complications.

2. Blood sugar is raised by:

> **a. food and drink, especially those containing carbohydrates;**
> **b. the patient's own liver (the liver stores and releases glucose);**
> **c. stress hormones;**
> **d. growth and sex hormones;**
> **e. some illnesses; and**
> **f. some medicines, including cortisone injections and steroids taken by mouth[3]**

---

[3] These are the most common factors which raise blood sugar. There are additional, less common factors which may also raise blood sugar in PWD (e.g., high altitude).

3. Symptoms of hyperglycemia are the same as the initial symptoms of Type 1 diabetes:

    a. **excessive thirst;**
    b. **frequent urination (sometimes seen as heavy diaper or bedwetting);**
    c. **increased appetite/ constant hunger;**
    d. **unexplained weight loss;**
    e. **blurry vision;**
    f. **fatigue/ tiredness; and**
    g. **irritability/ mood changes**

4. As described in Chapter 2, hyperglycemia which isn't treated can progress to diabetic ketoacidosis. People with T1D are at risk for DKA at any time, not just at diagnosis.

5. How to Treat a High Blood Sugar, as a general rule *(which does not apply to all people with Type 1 diabetes under all circumstances, so always follow your endocrinologist's personalized instructions)*:

    a. Check BG with a finger-stick to confirm a high blood sugar;
    b. Give insulin ***correction dose*** *(*aka ***correction bolus)*** according to the specific directions your endocrinologist has given you, making sure not to ***stack*** insulin (give insulin doses too close together in time, which is dangerous because it may cause a low blood sugar);
    c. Drink water;
    d. Check for ketones if BG is over 250 mg/dl;
    e. Exercise or walk if you can (but only if no ketones);
    f. Two hours after the insulin correction, check BG again; it should have gone down; and
    g. Call endo for instructions if, two hours after correcting, BG still hasn't decreased, or if patient has moderate or large ketones

<u>Summary</u>

- Hyperglycemia means high blood sugar.
- Food, the patient's own liver, hormones, some illnesses, and some medications raise blood sugar.
- Signs of high blood sugar include: extreme thirst, frequent urination, increased appetite/ constant hunger, unexplained weight loss, blurry vision, drowsiness/ fatigue, and irritability/ mood changes. People with T1D must always be on the lookout for hyperglycemia and should treat it according to their endocrinologist's directions.
- Hyperglycemia can progress to diabetic ketoacidosis (DKA), a life-threatening condition.
- Over the long term, poorly-controlled hyperglycemia can lead to serious medical complications.

Chapter 9

Hypoglycemia and
What Lowers Blood Sugar

> *When your blood sugar is dropping right before your family is going out to dinner: "One second, I just need to eat before we go out to eat."*
>
> *"I'm sorry for what I said when my blood sugar was low."*

1. *Hypoglycemia* **means low blood sugar -- too little glucose (sugar) in the blood. Insulin, exercise/ physical activity, and some illnesses lower blood sugar.**

A patient doesn't feel well when his blood sugar is too low. A very low blood sugar which is not treated can be life-threatening.

Generally, a blood sugar level less than 70 mg/dL is considered to be hypoglycemia. Severe hypoglycemia is the inability to treat oneself to raise blood sugar or a loss of consciousness.

2. Initial symptoms of hypoglycemia are:

    a. shakiness;
    b. anxiety/ nervousness;
    c. sweating/ clamminess/ chills;
    d. fast/ pounding heartbeat;
    e. irritability; and
    f. excessive hunger

3. If blood sugar is low and CONTINUES to fall, the brain doesn't get enough glucose. When this happens, additional symptoms of hypoglycemia may include:

    a. **difficulty concentrating;**
    b. **confusion;**
    c. **slurred speech;**
    d. **clumsiness/ lack of coordination;**
    e. **bizarre behavior; and**
    f. **tingling/ numbness in lips or tongue**

4. Finally, if blood sugar falls even further, a person with T1D may lose consciousness, have seizures, go into a coma, and, in rare instances, die.

5. People with Type 1 diabetes can often sense or feel their own low blood sugar. In the weeks and months after diagnosis, they will learn to recognize how they feel when their BG is low or is dropping quickly.

Over time, some patients lose the ability to feel their own lows. Not being able to feel one's own low blood sugar is called *hypoglycemia unawareness*. A person with Type 1 who can't feel his own low blood sugar won't know to test and treat it when he should. This potentially dangerous situation can be addressed by using a *continuous glucose monitor (CGM)* (see Chapter 13).

Some people with T1D have a *diabetes alert dog (DAD)*, a service dog which has been specifically trained to detect a low blood sugar and to alert the PWD and others to it.

6. How to Treat a Low Blood Sugar:

A low blood sugar should be treated as soon as possible to raise it back into the target range. As a general rule *(which does not apply to all people with Type 1 diabetes under all circumstances, so always follow your endocrinologist's personalized instructions),* **a low blood sugar should be treated as follows:**

a. If BG is below 70 mg/dL and person can eat, drink, and swallow:

(1) Consume 15 grams of a simple carbohydrate, such as apple juice or chewable glucose tablets. If you don't have juice or glucose tablets, treat the low with half of a standard 12-ounce can of regular soda, four level teaspoons of table sugar, or one tablespoon of honey.

Avoid treating a low blood sugar with desserts or junk food like ice cream, milkshakes, donuts, pizza, chocolate, candy bars, pie, cake, cookies, french fries, or chips. These foods contain fat, and will take longer to raise blood sugar than a simple carbohydrate with no fat.

Treating a low blood sugar with desserts and junk food can also form bad habits and cause unnecessary weight gain.

If a PWD is having a low blood sugar and there are no simple carbohydrates available to treat it, then by all means go ahead and treat the low with a dessert or junk food snack to raise BG.

(2) Wait 10-15 minutes, then test blood sugar again to make sure that it is in the target range.

If it is and if the next meal is more than one hour away, eat a protein snack to help stabilize blood sugar.

If you test and blood sugar is still not in the target range, treat again with another 15 grams of carbohydrate, wait another 10-15 minutes, and test again.

Treating a low with 15 grams of carbohydrate, waiting 15 minutes for it to raise blood sugar, then testing again is called the *Rule of 15*.

b. If BG is below 70 mg/dL and person is conscious, but can't eat, drink, or swallow:

(1) Someone must administer *glucagon*, a hormone used to raise blood sugar in cases of severe hypoglycemia. It is rare for glucagon to have to be used, but it is important that you always have unexpired glucagon and that you know where it is in case of emergency. Before administering any kind of glucagon, turn the

person on his side to prevent choking if he vomits. Glucagon kits currently come in three forms (mix and inject; auto-inject, and nasal glucagon), so follow the instructions on the particular glucagon kit you have.

(2) Wait 10-15 minutes and test blood sugar again. If the person's blood sugar hasn't risen to the target range, call 911.

c. If BG is below 70 mg/dL and person is unconscious:

Call 911. Turn person on his side and administer glucagon according to the instructions on the particular glucagon kit you are using.

T1D mom tip: There is an expiration date printed on every glucagon kit. In my personal calendar, on the date two weeks before the expiration date, I add: Refill glucagon kit before (expiration date).

T1D dad tip: Before I throw out expired "mix and inject" glucagon, I practice the steps required to give a glucagon injection.

Summary

- Hypoglycemia means low blood sugar (generally, less than 70 mg/dL).
- Insulin, activity, and certain illnesses can lower blood sugar.
- Initial symptoms of low blood sugar include: shakiness; anxiety/nervousness; sweating/clamminess/chills; fast/pounding heartbeat; irritability; and excessive hunger.
- If a low blood sugar continues to fall, additional symptoms may include: difficulty concentrating; confusion; slurred speech; clumsiness/ lack of coordination; bizarre behavior; and tingling/ numbness in lips or tongue.
- Treat a low blood sugar with a simple, fast-acting carbohydrate (such as apple juice or glucose tablets) if the person can swallow; if the person can't swallow or is unconscious, give glucagon.
- Severe hypoglycemia which is left untreated can cause seizure, coma, and, in rare instances, death.

Chapter 10

Diabetes Supplies

"I hate when I check my blood sugar and people ask me, "Doesn't that hurt?" I'm all, "Nooo, people with Type 1 diabetes don't feel any pain at all."

1. A person with Type 1 must always have easy access to her diabetes supplies.

2. At home, designate one place where you keep most of your diabetes supplies.

3. Children who attend school usually keep a second set of supplies in the school nurse's office. Many adults with T1D keep a second set of supplies at work.

4. When they are on the go, people with T1D must bring their supplies with them. They carry their supplies in bags (sometimes referred to as *diabetes bags*, diabetes kits, *D-bags*, or "go-bags") -- backpacks, drawstring/ cinch bags which can be worn as backpacks, satchels, handbags, sling bags, and waist packs (aka fanny packs or bum packs).

T1D mom tip: The school nurse keeps my daughter's diabetes supplies in her office in a clear plastic container with a lid, labeled with my daughter's name.

T1D dad tip: In case of a lockdown or a lockdown drill at my son's high school, we keep a box of emergency diabetes supplies in the teacher's desk in every classroom where he has a class.

5. The basic diabetes supplies are:

    a. ***Lancing Device*** and ***Lancets*** for doing a finger-stick to get a drop of blood to check blood sugar

        (1) It's important to have a clean fingertip when testing blood sugar. If possible, wash hands with soap and water before testing. If fingertips aren't clean, the BG readout may be inaccurate.

        (2) If using rubbing alcohol or hand sanitizer to clean the fingertip, don't use the first drop of blood to test BG because the product may distort the readout. Wipe away the first drop, then use the second drop of blood to test.

        (3) Discard a lancet after one use and replace it with a fresh lancet for the next use. The more a lancet is used, the duller the tip becomes, and the more it will hurt.

T1D dad tip: Stick the sides of the fingertips, not the tops or pads. The sides are less sensitive than the tops or pads. Rotate fingers so that you aren't always sticking the same spot or spots.

T1D mom tip: When doing a finger-stick, keep the hand down, below heart level, and gently "milk" the finger-stick to get a good, usable drop of blood.

T1D teen tip: At first, it hurt to do a finger-stick. After a few weeks, though, my fingertips became calloused and the finger-sticks didn't bother me as much.

    b. ***Meter*** (aka ***glucometer***) and compatible ***Test Strips*** to measure blood sugar levels

        (1) Today's meters require very little blood and are easy to use.

        (2) After opening the lid of a test strip container to get a test strip, make sure to close the lid again to protect the remaining test strips. Exposing them to light can affect their accuracy.

(3) Meters are powered by batteries or electricity. Remember to keep your meter powered.

(4) You may keep one meter at home and another at your school or office, but remember to bring all of the meters you use to your endocrinology appointments. Someone in the endo's office should also check the accuracy of your meters at every diabetes checkup.

(5) Meters keep a record of a user's blood sugar testing. At every appointment, this record will be reviewed. The endocrinologist will analyze the information and may use it to recommend changes to improve diabetes management.

CDE tip: The meter keeps a record of dates and times when the user has tested her blood sugar and the corresponding results. Sometimes, children and teens who have T1D will tell me that they test multiple times a day, but the meter shows that this is not true.

c. **Insulin** - the man-made prescription insulin(s) which people with T1D must inject or infuse every day (One notable exception is Afrezza, an inhalable insulin, but it is currently approved only for adults and only under certain conditions (see Chapter 27).

d. **Insulin Delivery Device** - a device used to deliver insulin into the body

(1) A PWD delivers insulin into her body by injection (with a ***syringe*** or insulin pen) or infusion from an insulin pump.

(2) Insulin is delivered ***subcutaneously*** (just beneath the skin), so that it can be slowly absorbed into the bloodstream. Don't inject insulin into a vein or muscle.

(3) Use a new needle for every injection. Reusing needles can result in infection or receiving the wrong dose of insulin.

(4) If you are new to giving injections, have someone else check that you are giving the right amount of insulin before you inject.

(5) When using an insulin pen, it's important to prime it before every injection. Priming pushes any air bubbles out of the pen so that the subsequent real injection will deliver the exact number of units desired.

(6) Like meters, insulin pumps keep records. Expect your endocrinologist to review information from your insulin pump at every endocrinology appointment.

T1D mom tip: When you inject with an insulin pen and have pressed the button to deliver insulin, count slowly to five before withdrawing the needle. This ensures delivery of the entire amount intended.

e. **Batteries** and/ or **Chargers** to power the devices that require them

f. **Food or drink to treat a low blood sugar** - It's best to use a simple carbohydrate like apple juice or chewable glucose tablets which will raise BG quickly.

g. ***Ketone Test Strips*** to test urine for the presence and size of ketones

h. **Glucagon** kit in case of an emergency low blood sugar

i. **Snack Food** to eat in case you have gone longer than you should without eating

*T1D mom tip: A 4 oz. serving of apple juice usually contains 15 grams of carbohydrates. Many of us **D-moms** buy cardboard juice boxes (each with an attached straw) for convenience. Make sure to check that the juice boxes you buy contain 4 oz. of juice; some contain more.*

j.   **Sharps box** is the special container you will keep at home to dispose of your used lancets, syringes, pen needles, test strips, and any other diabetes item which is sharp or which has any bodily fluids on it.

If you don't have a sharps box, contact your city or town to ask for disposal instructions for these items. Some municipalities, for example, will allow disposal in a hard plastic container (like a laundry detergent bottle) with a closed cap and a piece of tape with the handwritten message "Medical waste: Do Not Recycle" affixed.

Summary

- A person with Type 1 diabetes must always have quick access to her diabetes supplies, including a simple carbohydrate like apple juice or glucose tablets to treat a low blood sugar.
- Whenever a person with Type 1 goes anywhere, she must bring all of her diabetes supplies with her.
- Use a new lancet for every finger-stick and a new needle for every injection.

Chapter 11

Multiple Daily Injections;
Basal and Bolus Insulin

Basal -- it's not just a flavorful herb!

*Another parent: "I could never give my kid
a shot like that."*
*Me: "Yes, you could. I promise you, you could and
you would, without missing a beat. In the face of death,
needles are no big thing."*

1. Most people who have T1D begin treatment using *multiple daily injections* **(***MDIs,* **aka shots) to get insulin into their bodies.** Injections are given subcutaneously, i.e., just beneath the skin -- not intravenously (into a vein). MDIs are given with a syringe and needle or with an insulin pen (pen) and attached needle.

2. People who use multiple daily injections must use two different kinds of insulin -- *basal insulin* **and** *bolus insulin.*

    a. Basal insulin is sometimes called "background insulin" or "circulating insulin." A PWD must have basal insulin in his system at all times. Basal insulin helps keep blood glucose levels steady overnight and between meals.

For people on MDIs, basal insulin is usually a "long-acting" insulin which works in the body for up to 24 hours, or until the next basal injection is scheduled to be given. Basal insulin is usually injected once or twice a day. Your endo will tell you how much basal insulin to inject and when you should inject it.

<u>T1D mom tip</u>: I set a recurring alarm on my cell phone for 8 p.m., the time when my son is supposed to get his basal insulin injection. If he or I forget, the alarm reminds us.

> **b. Bolus insulin is insulin which is given to reduce increases in blood sugar from food or to correct a high blood sugar.**
>
> **Bolus insulin is injected whenever a patient eats a meal or snack which will raise his blood sugar.** Bolus insulin is usually "rapid-acting" insulin.
>
> When a PWD prepares to give himself his mealtime or snacktime bolus insulin, he simultaneously accounts for his correction dose. The correction dose is the amount of insulin required to lower his blood sugar level at that moment in time to his ***target blood glucose*** (determined in advance by his endocrinologist). Your diabetes team will teach you how to calculate bolus insulin doses for food and correction doses. The two doses are combined into one bolus injection. Again, these calculations are different for different people, so always follow the instructions which your endocrinologist has personalized for you.

3. Rapid-acting insulin begins to work approximately 10-20 minutes after injection, so it is recommended that people with T1D inject it 10-20 minutes before eating. Once injected, it remains active in the body for a total of approximately 4-5 hours.

As a general rule, a PWD who has a high blood sugar after he has injected bolus insulin and finished eating shouldn't give himself a correction dose injection until at least 2-3 hours after his last bolus injection. Injecting again before the 2-3 hour mark is stacking insulin and may lead to a low blood sugar. Ask your endocrinologist how long you should wait before giving a correction dose.

4. People who use multiple daily injections must rotate injection *sites* **(locations).** If insulin is injected at the same site repeatedly, scar tissue can build up. This scar tissue can interfere with insulin absorption and may also become cosmetically unattractive.

5. A common mistake made by those who do MDIs is mixing up basal insulin and bolus insulin when injecting. Try to avoid making this mistake, but if you do, contact your endo immediately for instructions on how to proceed.

T1D mom confession and tip: One night, I accidentally used the rapid-acting bolus insulin pen to inject my son instead of the long-acting basal insulin pen. I immediately called the endocrinologist, who advised me what I needed to do. From then on, I kept the basal insulin pen near my child's bed, and the bolus insulin pen in the kitchen, where my child eats.

Summary

- Those who use multiple daily injections must inject two different types of insulin every day -- basal insulin and bolus insulin.
- Basal insulin is the long-acting "background" insulin which people with T1D must have in their bodies at all times.
- Bolus insulin is the rapid-acting insulin used to reduce increases in blood sugar from food and to correct high blood sugar.

Chapter 12

Insulin Pumps

*"No, that's not a 'pager' clipped to my waistband.
It isn't 1980 anymore."*

*Some people wear their hearts on their sleeves.
I wear my pancreas on my waistband.*

1. An insulin pump is a computerized device which delivers insulin through a tiny *cannula* (flexible tube) or needle just beneath the skin. This method of delivering insulin into the body is called an infusion.

2. An insulin pump is NOT an implant. The pump itself remains outside the body.

3. Today's insulin pumps are small and lightweight. Most resemble small cell phones.

4. A pump eliminates the need for multiple daily injections because it infuses insulin under the skin 24 hours a day. A pump uses only rapid-acting insulin, and it uses it to deliver both basal and bolus insulin.

5. People with T1D who want to use an insulin pump must go through training to learn how to use a particular pump. All pump companies have a 24/7/365 toll-free "help line" you can call whenever you need help with your pump.

6. Your endocrinologist will give you personalized information to enter into your pump. Doing this is similar to the way you enter telephone numbers and other information into a smartphone. This information, the pump's settings, includes your ***insulin-to-carbohydrate ratio(s)***, basal insulin dose(s), target BG, and target range. Once the settings have been input, the pump will automatically do some of the math you have to do with MDIs. Always keep a copy of your pump's current settings.

7. Most pumps connect to an *infusion set* with very narrow tubing. It is the infusion set -- not the pump itself -- which attaches to the body. Insulin from the pump travels into the infusion set's very narrow tubing, and then into a cannula or thin needle just beneath the skin. (An exception is the OmniPod insulin pump. It is a tubeless pump which attaches directly to the outside of a patient's body and delivers insulin through an attached cannula just beneath the skin.)

8. A PWD who uses a pump must choose a site on her body where she will attach her infusion set (or her tubeless OmniPod pump). **Just as people who do multiple daily injections must rotate injection sites, a pump user must rotate infusion sites to avoid a buildup of scar tissue.**

9. Every two or three days, a *pumper* must replace her infusion set. To do so, she removes the infusion set attached to her body and replaces it with a new infusion set. At the same time, she refills her pump with new insulin. (In the case of the OmniPod, the entire pump is replaced every two or three days.)

10. Currently, an insulin pump requires the user to enter the number of grams of carbohydrate she is going to consume before it can deliver the correct bolus based on the user's personalized settings.

11. PWD keep their pumps in a variety of places. A pump can be clipped to the user's waistband or stored in a roomy pocket. A pump can be hidden under clothing in an insulin pump belt or undergarment specifically designed to hold insulin pumps. Pump holders and

accessories can be purchased online and come in different sizes, materials, and colors.

12. Some pumps are waterproof. Pumps which are not waterproof have a simple "disconnect" feature the person uses when she showers, bathes, or swims. Before getting wet, the user disconnects from the pump, but leaves the infusion set attached to her body. When she finishes her shower, bath or swim, she reconnects to the pump. A pump user can stay disconnected from her pump for up to one hour per day.

13. If you're thinking about getting an insulin pump, consider the user's age, ability, activities, and lifestyle, in addition to the general advantages and disadvantages of pumps:

    a. Advantages of a pump include:

        (1) No more multiple daily injections;
        (2) Less frequent low blood sugars;
        (3) Ability to adjust basal insulin to prevent low blood sugars during exercise or overnight;
        (4) Pump's bolus calculator function makes it easier to determine correct insulin doses;
        (5) More schedule flexibility;
        (6) More precise insulin delivery; and
        (7) Lower A1c

    b. Disadvantages of a pump include:

        (1) Must learn how to set the pump up, attach it to the body, and use it (more technical than injections);
        (2) Having a pump and/ or infusion set attached to the body day and night;
        (3) Having to decide where to keep the pump (may be affected by type of clothing and activity);
        (4) May be expensive if not fully covered by insurance;
        (5) Possible pump or infusion set problem, in which case the user (or the user's parent or caregiver) needs to be aware of the problem, and mature and competent enough to try to solve it;

(6) If the problem can't be solved promptly, the user must be prepared to use multiple daily injections until the problem is solved; and

(7) Pumpers who aren't getting proper insulin infusions can go into DKA sooner than those who do MDIs.

T1D mom tip: I used to have to give my daughter seven insulin injections a day. Going on a pump eliminated the need for those seven daily shots. With a pump, she gets only one needle stick every three days (when it is time to change her infusion set) to get insulin. That alone was a huge improvement -- for her and for me.

T1D tween tip: I'm on a pump all year long except during the summer, when I am on the swim team. Most days, I have to be in the pool for over an hour and my pump isn't waterproof, so I switch to multiple daily injections for the summer.

T1D child tip: I usually keep my pump in an insulin pump belt my mom bought on the Internet. It's very thin and stretchy and it has a pocket to hold my pump. I wear the belt under my clothes. You wouldn't know it's there if you looked at me. I even wear my pump belt under my pajamas when I sleep.

T1D adult tip: I keep my pump in my front pants pocket or in a special pump "holster" clipped to my waistband.

T1D teen tip: I love my pump and I would never voluntarily go back to multiple daily injections. It has really improved my quality of life.

T1D dad tip: My 13-year-old son was at a local amusement park with his friends when his pump battery died. He called me because he didn't have a replacement battery with him. I had him go to a store in the park, buy a AAA battery, and replace the bad battery in his pump.

T1D adult tip: I have used a pump for years, but I plan to go off it and use multiple daily injections on my wedding day. My diabetes team is giving me instructions on how to do that safely.

Summary

- An insulin pump is a small device which is attached to the outside of the body. It delivers insulin subcutaneously into the body 24 hours a day.
- A pump eliminates the need for multiple daily injections.
- There are advantages and disadvantages to using an insulin pump. Many factors should be considered in deciding whether a particular person should use a particular pump, including the user's age, ability, activities, lifestyle, and cost.

Chapter 13

Continuous Glucose Monitors

1. A person who has T1D must check his blood sugar many times a day. Most people with T1D check blood sugar with a finger-stick, test strip, and meter, which will display a blood sugar number.

2. A continuous glucose monitor (CGM) is another tool patients can use to check blood sugar. A CGM is a very small device with a tiny part (called a *sensor*) inserted just below the skin. The rest of the CGM sits above the skin. The sensor measures the user's blood sugar, and sends that measurement to a receiver (either a separate receiver device, a smartphone, or an insulin pump), which displays a blood sugar readout.

3. A CGM receiver displays a user's blood sugar level every few minutes, round-the-clock. Certain CGMs also show blood sugar *direction* (whether blood sugar is rising, falling, or staying about the same) and the *speed of increase or decrease* in blood sugar (how quickly or slowly blood sugar is rising or falling).

4. Some CGMs can be set to alert users with an audible alarm or a vibration. Alerts can also be silenced. CGM users specify the high and low blood sugar levels at which they would like to be alerted.

5. The information provided by CGMs is valuable because it lets a user know that he is having, or will soon have, a high or low blood sugar -- often before he can feel it on his own or confirm it with his meter. He can then take appropriate action. Doing so results in tighter control than he would have without a CGM.

6. Some CGMs have a "share" or "follow" feature which allows other people to receive blood sugar information about the CGM user on the other people's smart devices. If a child is wearing a CGM, his parents can see his blood sugar levels on their cell phones. Examples of times this would be especially helpful are in the middle of the night while the child is sleeping, while the child is at school, and when the child is at home with a babysitter.

7. A CGM can be used by those who use MDIs and those who use insulin pumps.

8. Blood sugar readings from a CGM and blood sugar readings from a meter are not usually identical, but they should be close. This is partly because a CGM's sensor measures *interstitial blood sugar* (from the interstitial fluid which surrounds cells), while a finger-stick measures blood sugar from the blood.

9. Until a few years ago, CGMs were not considered accurate enough to rely on for treatment decisions, so a user still had to do a finger-stick before making a treatment decision. Now, however, users of the *Dexcom G6* CGM and the *Freestyle Libre* CGM are allowed to make treatment decisions based on those CGMs' readouts without doing finger-sticks. Nonetheless, users are instructed to check BG with a finger-stick if symptoms do not correspond to a CGM's readout.

10. Some insulin pumps and CGMs work together as an integrated system in which the CGM communicates wirelessly with the wearer's insulin pump. If the CGM tells the pump that the user's blood sugar is -- or will soon become -- too high or too low, then the pump will

automatically adjust insulin delivery with the goal of getting the user's BG back in his target range. These systems are known as hybrid artificial pancreas systems.

T1D adult tip: When I was first diagnosed, the CGM technology wasn't anywhere near as good as it is today. Although I had a CGM then, there were so many false alarms that I stopped using it. Today, I use the Dexcom G6 and find it to be extremely accurate and reliable. Without my CGM, I wouldn't be able to keep such tight control.

T1D teen tip: Years ago, it hurt to attach the CGM to my body. The technology has improved so much since then that I can honestly say there is no pain at all when I attach my current CGM.

T1D mom tip: Getting my son a CGM was a game-changer for us. Being able to see his blood sugar numbers on my smartphone has reduced my anxiety a lot.

Summary

- A continuous glucose monitor (CGM) is a small device which a PWD attaches to the outside of his body. The CGM has a tiny sensor which is placed just below the skin and measures the user's blood sugar.
- A CGM is helpful because it provides information about blood sugar levels, trends, and rates (often before a user can feel a low or high blood sugar on his own) and enables the user to take prompt, appropriate action.
- The follow/ share feature on some CGMs allows parents and others to see the user's blood sugar levels.

Chapter 14

Complications and How to Reduce Risk

My relationship status with Type 1 diabetes:
Not Complicated

1. Complications are the serious -- sometimes even life-threatening -- long-term health problems which people with T1D may develop as a result of years of poorly-controlled blood sugar. While complications may develop, they are NOT inevitable. Today, if a person with Type 1 puts in the effort to correctly manage her diabetes, she will dramatically reduce her risk of developing complications, and may never have any diabetes-related complications at all.

2. Complications develop cumulatively over time. Poorly-controlled high blood sugar damages blood vessels in the heart, legs, feet, eyes, kidneys, and nerves. This damage may eventually lead to kidney failure, blindness, nerve damage, amputation, heart disease, and stroke. **Patients don't feel the damage to their blood vessels while it's taking place. It's only after years of uncontrolled high blood sugar that complications appear.** Diabetes does damage which is usually not visible or noticeable until it's too late.

3. It can be very upsetting to learn about complications, but you should take comfort in the knowledge that current treatments for T1D are much better than they were in the past -- and will undoubtedly be even better in the future. Don't assume that a person with Type 1 diabetes diagnosed today will have the same complications which people with T1D diagnosed decades ago had or have.

4. Up until the early 1990s, the standard treatment for Type 1 diabetes was only one or two insulin injections a day.

5. In 1993, a landmark scientific study called the Diabetes Control and Complications Trial (the DCCT) changed the way diabetes was treated. (See Chapter 7 for more detailed information about the DCCT.)

The DCCT proved that intensive treatment (close monitoring of BG levels, multiple daily injections or infusions, and frequent checkups with a patient's diabetes team) **was better than the standard treatment which most people with T1D followed before the DCCT. Intensive treatment led to tighter control of blood sugar, and was found to:**

    a. **lower A1c;**
    b. **dramatically reduce the risk of complications from diabetes; and**
    c. **slow the progression of any existing complications**

6. Although intensive treatment (aka intensive management) takes more time and effort, the outcomes are much better than they were with the standard treatment recommended for people with T1D before the DCCT.

A person with T1D who puts in the time and effort of intensive management will have tighter control of blood sugar, allowing her to live a longer and healthier life. It's even possible that she may never have any complications from T1D.

Summary

- Complications are the serious health problems which people with Type 1 diabetes may develop after years of poorly-controlled high blood sugar.
- Intensive treatment of T1D lowers A1c and dramatically reduces the risk of complications from T1D.

Chapter 15

Food and Diet; Counting Carbohydrates

Things a Person with Type 1 Diabetes Cannot Eat:
1. Poison
2. Cookies with Poison

"Now, before we carve the turkey, let's "SWAG"
(make a "scientific wild-ass guess")
how many carbs are in the stuffing!"

In math class, I was THAT person who repeatedly asked
when we were ever going to use the stuff they were
teaching us. The joke was on me, though, because
as the father of a child with Type 1 diabetes,
I use math every single day.

1. Food contains three types of nutrients: *protein, fat,* and *carbohydrate.* A person needs food containing *all three* of these nutrients to be healthy.

   a. Foods containing *protein* include meats, poultry, fish, eggs, cheese, and tofu.
   b. Foods containing *fat* include oils, butter, margarine, mayonnaise, cream, salad dressing, avocados, and peanut butter.
   c. Foods containing *carbohydrate* (*carbs*) include bread, crackers, cereal, rice, pasta, grains, milk, yogurt, fruit, fruit juice, starchy vegetables like corn, peas, potatoes and beans, cake, pie, ice cream, other desserts, chips, pretzels, regular soft drinks, sports drinks, and other sweetened drinks.

2. The nutrient which has the greatest effect on blood sugar levels is the carbohydrate. Consuming food or drink which contains more than a negligible amount of carbohydrate will raise blood sugar.

This does NOT mean that all carbohydrates are bad for people with T1D. Carbohydrates provide the body with energy. Many foods containing carbohydrates also contain important vitamins and minerals.

When discussing foods with carbohydrates, **it's important to distinguish between healthy and unhealthy foods.** Some foods containing carbs are better, healthier choices than others. An apple and a single serving of regular potato chips may each contain the exact same quantity of carbohydrate, but the potato chips are an unhealthy food choice because they are a processed food, high in calories, often contain unhealthy trans-fat and/ or saturated fat, are high in sodium, are low in vitamins and minerals, and have almost no fiber. By contrast, the apple is a healthy food choice because it is an unprocessed whole food and contains vitamins, minerals, antioxidants, and fiber.

3. Generations ago, people with T1D were told to avoid foods containing table sugar (sucrose) because it was believed that sugar itself was mainly responsible for raising blood sugar. This turned out not to be entirely true. **In fact, it was not *JUST* sugar, but more broadly, foods containing carbohydrates which raise blood sugar.**

4. Another discovery was that insulin could be given to PWD based on the amount of carbohydrate consumed and the patient's unique insulin needs. These discoveries meant that people with Type 1 no longer had to completely avoid foods containing sugar.

5. Today, there is no such thing as a "diabetes diet." Nor is a person who has T1D limited to special foods or a complicated diet plan. Like everyone else, a person with Type 1 diabetes should strive for a balanced, heart-healthy diet.

A balanced, heart-healthy diet means:

    a. eating fruits and vegetables, complex carbohydrates, and lean proteins;

    b. limiting processed foods like junk food, sweets, foods with added sugar, sweetened drinks, and alcohol;

    c. avoiding trans-fats and limiting foods high in saturated fat;

    d. choosing unsaturated fats;

    e. eating portioned amounts; and

    f. achieving or maintaining a healthy weight

6. You may hear the statement: "A person with Type 1 diabetes can eat anything he wants." This is true in the sense that today, no food is completely forbidden for people with Type 1. The statement, however, is not a "pass" for people with T1D to ignore healthy eating.

"A person with Type 1 diabetes *CAN* eat anything he wants" does NOT mean that he *SHOULD* eat anything he wants AT ANY TIME. As an example, a PWD should not eat donuts every day for breakfast.

"A person with Type 1 diabetes *CAN* eat anything he wants" does NOT mean that portion size doesn't matter. It does matter.

7. At every age and stage of life, a person with T1D has specific dietary requirements, just like his counterparts who don't have T1D. Dietary needs and insulin needs often change as a PWD grows and develops. A registered dietitian can work with you to create a healthy eating plan based on your age, weight, physical activity, food preferences, and lifestyle.

8. Before a PWD eats any snack or meal, he has to determine how many grams of carbohydrate are in that snack or meal.[4] This is called ***counting carbohydrates,*** or simply, ***counting carbs***. Every person who is expected to count carbs for himself or for a child or loved one should attend a carb-

---

[4] Sometimes, newly-diagnosed patients are taught about the "food exchange system" and are given personalized "sliding scales" to use to match the food they eat to the insulin they will need. Most people with Type 1, however, soon match the food they eat to insulin by counting carbohydrates and using their own personalized insulin-to-carbohydrate ratios.

counting class. At first, counting carbohydrates is difficult, but -- as with any new challenge -- the more you do it, the easier it will become. After a few weeks or months, counting carbs will be one of your new skills.

T1D dad confession: When I first heard that I would have to figure out how many carbs were in any meal or snack my son was going to eat, it seemed like I would never be able to do it. I attended a carb-counting class, where I was given the Calorie King book. I also downloaded the My Fitness Pal app to my phone. At home, I used a food scale, a measuring cup, and a measuring spoon. It was hard at first, but after a month or so, I felt comfortable counting carbs.

T1D adult tip: I've learned that I can't always rely on the nutrition information on restaurants' websites. That information corresponds to a particular food, prepared a particular way, in a particular quantity, in a food laboratory. The restaurant where I'm eating may not reproduce the dish the exact same way. I use restaurant nutrition information as a starting point, but also use my carb-counting skills if the nutrition information provided doesn't seem right or could be off.

T1D mom tip: When we started counting carbs, I always used a book or app to figure out the carb count. Six months later, I knew dozens of foods' carb counts by heart.

9. A PWD should have a food scale, measuring cups, and measuring spoons to weigh and measure food before eating. Unless the food you eat has a nutrition label which states how many grams of carbohydrate are in the exact portion of food you will eat, weighing and measuring food before you eat it is the best way to determine how many carbohydrates a portion of food contains. Remember: **Portion size matters when counting carbs.**

10. When counting carbs, pay attention to the "form" of the food when it will be eaten. For example, the nutrition label on a package of dry rice may state that one cup of rice contains 40 grams of carbohydrate, but does this information refer to one cup of dry, uncooked rice or one cup of cooked rice? The answer is important because one cup of dry rice contains many more grams of carbohydrate than one cup of cooked rice. Examine the

nutrition label to check if it specifies the form of the food (e.g., dry vs. cooked). If it doesn't, consult another reliable source for the answer.

11. Once a PWD determines how many grams of carbohydrate he's going to eat, he uses that information to determine how much insulin he's going to need to *cover the carbohydrates* (account for the carbohydrate intake with insulin).
The amount of insulin needed depends on several factors, including the individual's personal insulin-to-carbohydrate ratio.

12. Your endocrinologist will tell you what your personal insulin-to-carb ratio is. Insulin-to-carb ratio means that 1 unit of insulin will cover a certain number of grams of carbohydrate consumed. For example, if an endocrinologist tells her patient that his insulin-to-carb ratio is 1 to 10, (usually written "1:10"), this means that the patient should give himself 1 unit of insulin for every 10 grams of carbohydrate he consumes.
Every person with T1D has his own unique insulin-to-carb ratio. Some patients have different insulin-to-carb ratios for different times of the day. A patient's insulin-to-carb ratio(s) may also change over time.

13. Make sure that you understand the insulin-to-carb ratio and how to determine the correct amount of insulin needed for snacks and meals. If you are unsure, ask a member of your diabetes team to review it with you until you do understand. **Giving too much insulin will result in low blood sugar. Giving too little insulin will result in high blood sugar.**

14. It's still a common misconception that people with T1D shouldn't eat foods or drinks containing sugar. People with T1D may eat foods and drinks containing sugar, as long as they make sure to take the appropriate amount of insulin to cover the carbs.

15. It's also a common misconception that PWD should eat only "sugar-free" or "no sugar added" foods. "Sugar-free" and "no sugar added" DO NOT NECESSARILY MEAN "carb-free." If there are carbs in "sugar-free" or "no sugar added" foods, those foods are likely to raise blood sugar, and insulin must still be given.

16. It's safe for PWD to use artificial sweeteners such as Splenda, Sweet 'n Low, and Equal, which don't raise blood sugar. Some packaged foods contain "sugar alcohols," which will be listed on the nutrition label under ingredients. Although sugar alcohols won't raise BG, they may lead to gastrointestinal problems (bloating, gas and diarrhea). If you consume foods with sugar alcohols, make sure to limit the portion size.

T1D mom tip: When my daughter was diagnosed, I decided that everyone in the family was going to eat the same meals. I didn't want my daughter to see her non-T1D brother eating foods which I wasn't serving to her. My entire family eats much healthier now.

T1D dad tip: When I pack my 8th grade son's lunch, I enclose a piece of paper with the names of the foods I've included and the corresponding carb counts. I include a total carb count, which he uses if he's going to eat everything I've packed. If he wants to eat less, he can add up the carbs of the items he wants to eat and dose his insulin off of that carb count.

T1D adult tip: I've learned that complex carbohydrates don't spike my blood sugar like simple carbohydrates do. When I ate white toast (a simple carbohydrate) for breakfast, my blood sugar would spike, I wouldn't feel well, and I had to wait at least two hours to correct. Now I eat oatmeal (a complex carbohydrate) for breakfast. Complex carbohydrates take longer for the body to break down into glucose. The glucose enters my system more slowly and gives me a steady flow of energy, keeping my blood sugar on a more even keel.

T1D grandmother tip: It's a myth that people who have T1D can't eat desserts or sweets. They can eat anything, including desserts, as long as they figure out the carb count and take the appropriate amount of insulin.

T1D mom tip: Once my daughter was diagnosed, I began paying much closer attention to the food our family ate. I stopped buying junk food and focused on healthy, tasty foods. I also prepare healthier meals (or order healthy meals if we eat out). We still have dessert, but we try to limit the frequency to three times a week, and we also limit the portion size. My entire family is benefiting from healthier eating. I myself lost ten pounds in the first three months after my daughter's diagnosis.

<u>T1D dad tip</u>: We don't put any restrictions on what our child eats on special occasions like his birthday or Thanksgiving. At those times, we just make sure to cover the carbs.

<u>T1D mom tip</u>: My daughter doesn't require insulin for snacks with less than 10 grams of carbohydrate. I always keep snacks in the house which have less than 10 grams of carbs (like sugar-free Jell-O, celery sticks, string cheese, and turkey breast) so that she can snack without having to inject insulin.

<u>T1D mom tip</u>: It's important to remember that portion size matters when counting carbs. One day, my eight-year-old son asked me if he could have a breath mint from my handbag. I said yes, but first he needed to check the carb count on the label. He did, and told me that it was one gram of carbohydrate. I said that he could eat it without injecting. Well … little did I know that he would eat twenty mints! The serving size on the label was for one mint! This meant that he consumed 20 grams of carbohydrate without taking any insulin for it. Needless to say, his blood sugar rose and we had to correct it.

<u>Summary</u>

- Like everyone, people with Type 1 diabetes should eat a healthy, well-balanced diet.
- It's a popular misconception that people with T1D cannot eat foods containing sugar.
- The nutrient in food which raises blood sugar the most is the carbohydrate.
- People with Type 1 must determine the amount of carbohydrate in all food and drink they consume, and dose the correct amount of insulin for them to "cover" those carbs.
- "Sugar-free" foods are not necessarily recommended for people with T1D. Even if a food is "sugar-free," it may not be "carb-free."

Chapter 16

Sick Days; Medical Procedures and Surgery

> *Lucky me! I have an illness on top of my chronic illness!*

1. Like everyone, PWD occasionally become sick with illnesses such as the common cold, flu, or stomach bug, or have symptoms such as fever, vomiting, or diarrhea.

2. **When a person with T1D is sick, she must still take care of her diabetes. In fact, she must be extra careful with diabetes management on sick days, because illness can also affect blood sugar.**

3. **When a PWD is sick, test her blood sugar and check her urine for ketones every 2 - 3 hours. Be aware that illness can lead to DKA. Keep her hydrated because dehydration raises the risk of DKA. If she has moderate or large ketones, call the endo for advice.**

4. **People with T1D need insulin even on sick days. Make sure to take the usual dose of long-acting or basal insulin. Take bolus insulin to cover the carbs in the food and drink consumed.**

5. **Sometimes, being sick will make blood sugar rise.** In response to illness, the body may release stress hormones, which raise blood sugar. If blood sugar is high, drink water, sugar-free beverages, or broth. Eat if you can, and give bolus insulin to cover the carbs. Correct high BG as you've been instructed to do.

6. **Other times, being sick will make blood sugar fall.** A stomach bug which causes vomiting or diarrhea may lower blood sugar. Eat if you can, and give bolus insulin to cover the carbs. If blood sugar is low and you can't eat, drink beverages with sugar to prevent hypoglycemia. Treat low BG as you've been instructed to do.

7. Some medications, notably steroids like cortisone, raise BG. This doesn't mean that a PWD cannot take steroids if needed. It just means that her insulin dose may need to be raised to account for the steroid's effect on blood sugar.

8. Many over-the-counter medicines (including regular cough drops and regular cough syrup) contain carbs and may also raise blood glucose. Look for carb-free or low-carb alternatives to those which are high in carbs.

9. There may be times when a person with Type 1 will not be allowed to eat for a certain period of time, e.g., before a scheduled surgery, before a tooth extraction, or before getting braces put on. In these cases, tell the provider well in advance that the patient has Type 1 diabetes and needs to be scheduled for the first appointment of the morning.

In addition, tell your diabetes team in advance about the procedure because they may modify the patient's insulin dose up to 24 hours before the procedure.

10. Having Type 1 diabetes alone doesn't put a person at higher risk for other illnesses like cold and flu. Poorly-controlled T1D, however, weakens the immune system, and having a weakened immune system does increase one's risk of cold, flu, and other illnesses.

11. It's important for people with T1D to stay up to date on recommended immunizations, including getting an annual flu shot, to prevent illness.

Summary

- A PWD who is sick has to deal not only with the symptoms of that particular illness, but also with the effect that the illness has on her blood sugar.
- Some illnesses raise BG, while other illnesses lower BG.
- On sick days, a person with T1D still needs basal insulin and bolus insulin to cover carbs. Don't skip insulin on sick days.
- When a person with Type 1 is sick, she or her caregiver must frequently test blood sugar and check for ketones because illness can lead to DKA.

Chapter 17

Exercise and Physical Activity

1. Regular exercise is an important part of staying healthy for everyone, including people with Type 1 diabetes. It is recommended that people with T1D do at least 30 minutes of exercise, five days a week. Exercise has physical benefits (including strengthening the heart), emotional benefits (including reducing stress), and helps to maintain or lose weight.

2. Aerobic exercise (e.g., running, swimming, and playing soccer) lowers blood sugar in people with Type 1.

3. Some physical activities which aren't always thought of as exercise will also lower blood sugar. Examples are mowing the lawn, painting a room, and dancing.

4. The more demanding the exercise or physical activity, the more it will lower blood sugar. Running for 10 minutes will lower blood sugar more than walking for 10 minutes.

5. A person with T1D should anticipate that his blood sugar will fall during exercise, and can take precautions to prevent it from happening. Some people eat a snack with protein and carbs before they exercise and don't cover the carbs with insulin. Those who have pumps can temporarily reduce basal insulin delivery so that they get less insulin while exercising. Exercise's effect on blood sugar is highly individual and depends on many factors. PWD often use the "trial and error" method until they find what works for them.

6. Monitor BG before, during and after exercise. Exercise affects BG during exercise and sometimes also for hours afterwards. Make sure you have your diabetes supplies with you and be prepared to treat a low blood sugar. Wear your diabetes identification bracelet so that someone can identify you as a person with T1D in case you need help.

7. Keep in mind that stress hormones can cause blood sugar to rise. Some people with T1D report a temporary increase in blood sugar from stress hormones when they are nervous or excited before competitions.

8. Having Type 1 does not mean that you can't participate in sports or even be a competitive athlete. There are people of all ages with T1D in amateur, school, college, Olympic, and professional sports (see Chapter 30).

T1D dad tip: My son tested his blood sugar before he began hockey practice, and his meter read 85 mg/dl. He knew that if he wasn't proactive before he went on the ice, his blood sugar would drop, making him hypoglycemic. He ate a snack containing protein and 30 grams of carbohydrates, and purposely didn't give himself insulin to cover the carbs. He did this because he knew that the snack would raise his blood sugar, while the exercise would lower his blood sugar, and hopefully, he'd stay in his target range.

T1D athlete tip: I'm a competitive soccer player and I always test my blood sugar before I compete. I'm often a little higher than my target range, but I know that this is because I am nervous and excited about the match and my body has released stress hormones, which raise blood sugar. I also know that once I begin playing soccer, the exercise will lower my blood sugar.

T1D mom tip: A few weeks after my 15-year-old son was diagnosed, he and I painted his bedroom walls using long-handled rollers. Half an hour into painting, my son said that he was feeling low. He checked his blood sugar, and, sure enough, it was low. Before we started, we didn't think of painting as "exercise," but we realized that it is a physical activity and it did lower his blood sugar.

Summary

- It's very important for people with T1D to get regular exercise.
- Since exercise can affect blood sugar, a person with Type 1 must monitor BG before, during, and after exercise.
- A PWD may want to be proactive before he begins to exercise by eating an uncovered snack or temporarily lowering his basal insulin delivery from his pump.
- When a person with T1D exercises, he should always have his diabetes supplies nearby and should always be prepared to treat a low blood sugar.

Chapter 18

Sexuality and Pregnancy

> *"Yes, I CAN have children in spite of my Type 1 diabetes.
> Surprisingly, your obvious rudeness didn't prevent you
> from doing the same."*

1. People with Type 1 diabetes can certainly be intimate, have normal sex lives, and have healthy babies.

2. Sex is a physical activity and may lower blood sugar.

3. Test blood sugar before and after sex. Make sure that you have your diabetes supplies nearby, including something to treat a low blood sugar.

4. Your partner should know that you have Type 1 in case you need help.

5. For those on multiple daily injections, there is no "hardware" which might get in the way during intimacy.

6. Although it's possible to have sex while wearing an insulin pump, some people who use pumps choose to disconnect from their insulin pumps during sex. (This does not apply to the OmniPod insulin pump, which cannot be disconnected and reconnected like other pumps.) A PWD shouldn't stay disconnected from her pump for more than one hour per day, though, so it's important to remember to reconnect to the pump afterwards.

7. People who use multiple daily injections and those who use insulin pumps may also have continuous glucose monitors (CGMs) attached to their bodies. CGMs are smaller than pumps and shouldn't interfere with sex, so there is no need to remove them.

8. Always use birth control if you are not trying to become pregnant.

9. Ideally, a woman with Type 1 who wants to become pregnant should have her blood sugar under tight control before she even tries to conceive. Before she stops using birth control, she should consult her endocrinologist and obstetrician for special advice on diabetes management and blood sugar control before conception. The best outcomes with T1D pregnancies are those in which BG goals have been achieved before conception.

10. A woman with T1D should maintain tight blood sugar control throughout her pregnancy. She should be cared for by an obstetrician who is part of a maternal fetal medicine team, and will work in conjunction with her endocrinologist before, during, and after pregnancy. Her insulin needs will change throughout the pregnancy, and she will need her endo's ongoing advice to adjust insulin levels.

11. Poorly-controlled Type 1 diabetes increases the risks for mother and baby, including the risk of birth defects, miscarriage, and pre-term delivery.

12. Although having a mother or father with T1D increases a child's risk of developing the disease, it is still very unlikely that the child herself will develop T1D.

Summary

- People with Type 1 diabetes can have normal sex lives and healthy pregnancies.
- Ideally, a person with T1D should plan her pregnancy. She should meet certain blood sugar goals before conception and should keep tight control throughout the pregnancy.
- Not managing Type 1 diabetes appropriately before and during pregnancy increases the chances of undesirable outcomes for mother and baby.

Chapter 19

Alcohol

Talented as it is, my liver simply can't multi-task.

1. For several reasons, drinking alcohol is more dangerous for people with Type 1 diabetes than it is for those who don't have it.

2. First, glucagon (used to raise a very low blood sugar when a person with Type 1 is unconscious, or is conscious, but cannot eat, drink or swallow) will NOT work while the liver is busy metabolizing alcohol. Glucagon works by stimulating the liver to release the glucose it naturally stores. The liver, however, can't metabolize alcohol and release glucose at the same time. It therefore delays its job of releasing stored glucose while it is busy metabolizing alcohol.

3. Second, a low blood sugar can be mistaken for intoxication. When a PWD's blood sugar is very low, he may seem confused, incoherent, clumsy, or uncoordinated. His behavior may be bizarre. His speech may be slurred. Others who observe these strange behaviors may assume that the PWD is drunk, when in fact, he may *NOT* be drunk, but may be having a very low blood sugar. When others mistakenly believe that a person with T1D is drunk, they may not get him the appropriate help he needs to treat the low blood sugar. Left untreated, a low blood sugar which continues to fall can lead to seizure, coma, and, in rare instances, death.

4. Type 1 diabetes treatment is highly personalized, so before you drink any alcohol, ask your diabetes team for personalized advice about whether and how you can drink safely.

5. Alcoholic drinks tend to initially spike blood sugar, then lower it dramatically. People with T1D should be aware of this effect. Some PWD proactively take one or more of the following actions before they start drinking to help protect themselves from an alcohol-induced low blood sugar:

    a. Before drinking, eat a snack containing carbs, but don't cover the carbs with insulin;

    b. Choose an alcoholic drink low in carbs because it will have less of an effect on blood sugar. Keep in mind that some alcoholic drinks contain regular soda, fruit juice, or mixers, which are high in carbs;

    c. Don't give insulin for the first alcoholic drink; and

    d. Set a temporary basal on your insulin pump so that you will get less basal insulin than usual for a specified period of time.

6. Never drink on an empty stomach and always drink in moderation.

7. Test blood sugar before, during, and after drinking. Alcohol can affect blood glucose levels for up to 24 hours. If you've been drinking and you go to sleep, set an alarm to wake you up in a few hours to check your blood sugar, or make sure that your CGM alarms are on.

8. If you choose to drink alcohol, be prepared. Have all your diabetes supplies with you and make sure that the person you are with knows that you have T1D and what to do if you need help or are in an emergency situation.

Summary

- Alcohol poses special risks for people with Type 1 diabetes.
- Glucagon will not work while a PWD's liver is metabolizing alcohol.
- While most people with T1D can drink alcohol, they should take certain precautions before, during, and after drinking alcohol to stay safe.

Chapter 20

Smoking and Vaping

"Sure, I'll buy a pack for you. Do you prefer "emphysema lights" or "heart disease with menthol"?"

1. People who have Type 1 diabetes, like everyone else, should not smoke cigarettes or cigars. Smoking causes lung cancer, other cancers, and lung disease. It also damages the heart and blood vessels, increasing the risk of heart disease and stroke. Secondhand smoke causes the same disease and damage, so people with T1D should not be exposed to secondhand smoke.

2. Over time, poorly-controlled Type 1 damages blood vessels. This means that PWD have an increased risk of heart attack and stroke even if they don't smoke. When a PWD smokes, she further damages these blood vessels.

3. Electronic cigarette (e-cigarette) use (aka vaping) is relatively new and there is still a lot about it which is unknown. It has, however, been associated with severe lung disease. Supporters of e-cigarettes contend that vaping is less dangerous than traditional smoking. Even if future scientific studies support this claim, "less dangerous" doesn't necessarily mean that vaping is safe. Until we know more, federal and state authorities recommend avoiding all vaping. **People with T1D should therefore avoid vaping and the secondhand smoke that comes from it.**

Summary

People with T1D should not smoke cigarettes or cigars, or use electronic cigarettes.

Chapter 21

Driving

A new T1D low: having your driver's license revoked because you drove with a low blood sugar and caused an accident

1. Like other drivers, PWD have a legal and moral duty to drive safely and protect themselves, other drivers, passengers, pedestrians, and property.

2. **A person with T1D can certainly drive a car, but he should do so only when his blood sugar is in his target range. While driving with low blood sugar is more risky than driving with high blood sugar, high blood sugar can also interfere with driving skills.** Driving a car with either hypoglycemia or hyperglycemia can cause a serious accident.

3. **A person with Type 1 should check his blood sugar every time he gets behind the wheel to drive.** If he is hypoglycemic, he should treat his low, wait, and confirm that his blood sugar is in the target range before he starts to drive. If he is hyperglycemic, he should give himself a correction bolus and wait until his blood sugar is in his target range before he begins to drive.

4. **On long drives, every hour, a person with T1D should safely pull the car off the road to test his blood sugar.** Of course, if he feels or is alerted by his continuous glucose monitor that his blood sugar is low or going low before the one-hour mark, he should safely pull the car off the road and test at that time.

5. When driving, PWD should keep glucose tablets or juice boxes within easy reach to treat low blood sugars. Make sure to restock the car so that there is always enough product available to treat lows.

6. While laws on driving with T1D differ from state to state, all states want to make sure that licensed drivers don't pose a significant danger to themselves or others. A driver's license application usually asks if the applicant has "Type 1 diabetes," "diabetes," or another medical condition which might cause loss of consciousness or interfere with safe driving. Some states require a doctor's letter stating that the applicant's blood glucose control is good enough to drive safely. States may revoke, suspend, or restrict the driver's license of a PWD who has lied on his application or driven unsafely because of his diabetes. States also accept reports from physicians, hospitals, police officers, family members, and even anonymous sources about drivers with T1D who shouldn't be driving because of poor glucose control.

7. If a PWD is in a car accident, he may require medical attention. First responders and health care providers need to know if a person has Type 1 in order to treat him properly. For this reason, **a PWD should always wear a medical ID bracelet or a similar type of medical identification.**

<u>Summary</u>

A person with T1D should drive only when his blood glucose is within his target range, and should take other precautions to keep himself, other drivers, passengers, pedestrians, and property as safe as possible.

Chapter 22

Medical Identification (ID) Bracelets

Julia liked her medical ID bracelet so much that she decided to get the matching necklace and earrings.

1. People who have Type 1 diabetes are insulin-dependent, so it is vital for first responders, health care professionals, and others to be able to discover this quickly and easily in emergency situations.

2. Traditionally, PWD have been told to wear medical identification bracelets. In emergencies, first responders and health care providers are most likely to check people's wrists for medical ID bracelets.

At a minimum, a medical ID bracelet should identify the wearer as a person with Type 1 diabetes. Some people also include: the person's name; the words "insulin," "insulin-dependent," or "insulin pump," if applicable; and the name and telephone number of an emergency contact.

3. Instead of bracelets, some people with T1D wear medical ID "dog tag" necklaces or get tattoos identifying them as having Type 1 diabetes.

4. While not a replacement for a medical ID bracelet, dog tag necklace, or tattoo, it's also a good idea to carry a card in your wallet or backpack which identifies you as a person with Type 1 diabetes.

T1D dad tip: *My 8-year-old son wears the silicone "TYPE 1 DIABETES" bracelet he was given in the hospital when he was first diagnosed. It's waterproof and comfortable, so he never has to take it off.*

T1D mom tip: *My 16-year-old daughter didn't want to advertise to the world that she had Type 1. We let her choose a silver cuff bracelet from the Etsy website, and had it engraved "Type 1 Diabetes" on the face, and her emergency contact's phone number on the reverse side.*

T1D adult tip: *Before I went to college, I had "Type 1 Diabetes" tattooed on my wrist. This means that I never have to remember to wear a medical ID bracelet. It was also the only tattoo my parents were okay with me getting.*

T1D adult tip: *I wore a medical ID bracelet until I discovered a "watchband sleeve" which says "Type 1 Diabetes." I wear the sleeve on my smartwatch every day.*

Summary

A person with T1D should always wear a medical identification bracelet or have another item clearly identifying her as having Type 1 diabetes in case of emergency.

Chapter 23

T1D in School; 504 Plans and Accommodations; The School Nurse

---

*"Gave myself my insulin shot yesterday in class
& the girl next [to] me said "can you like not do
that right now"
um no Debra I'd like to live thx"*

(actual 2018 tweet by Meredith Barnes, college student with T1D)

---

1. When a child is diagnosed with Type 1 diabetes, his parents should notify his school counselor about the diagnosis as soon as possible. The parent should also ask the school counselor to notify all of the child's teachers, coaches, and the school nurse about the diagnosis. It is important for teachers and coaches to know what is going on so that they understand why the child is absent and that certain accommodations will be made once the child returns to school.

2. Two federal laws -- *Section 504 of the Rehabilitation Act of 1973 (Section 504)* and the *Americans with Disabilities Act (ADA)* -- cover children with Type 1 diabetes in virtually all elementary, middle, and high schools and colleges in the country.

3. Type 1 diabetes is considered to be a *disability* under these laws. Sometimes, PWD and their caregivers object to the word *disability* because they don't think of Type 1 as a disability. The meaning of "disability" under these specific laws, however, is different from the meaning of "disability" in ordinary language. Because Type 1 diabetes is considered to be a disability *under these particular laws*, students with Type 1 are entitled to certain legal protections.

4. In virtually all elementary, middle, and high schools, children with T1D have the right to enroll and participate. They also have the right to have trained school staff give them the T1D care they need to be safe. **Specifically, trained school staff should be able to:**

    a.   know and recognize the warning signs of hypoglycemia (low blood sugar);
    b.   know and recognize the warning signs of hyperglycemia (high blood sugar);
    c.   test blood sugar;
    d.   give insulin;
    e.   give glucagon; and
    f.   know how and when to get help

5. A *504 plan* (named for the Section 504 law) for a student with T1D is a written document listing the *accommodations* (special rules/ modifications of general school rules) applicable to that student at school so that he has the same access to education as other children, is treated fairly, and is medically safe.

A student who has T1D doesn't have to be struggling in school to get a 504 plan; having Type 1 diabetes alone means that a student is legally entitled to have a 504 plan.

6. There is no "one-size-fits-all" 504 plan for students with T1D because each student's 504 plan should be personalized for his specific needs. Nonetheless, some typical provisions in 504 plans are:

    a.   Teachers, coaches, bus drivers, and other school staff who have regular interaction with the student know how to recognize hypoglycemia and hyperglycemia and how to respond appropriately;
    b.   Multiple school staff members are trained to assist with T1D management, including checking blood glucose levels and administering insulin and glucagon;
    c.   Permission for student to go to the bathroom or water fountain when necessary;
    d.   Permission for student to eat when necessary;

e. Excused absences for endocrinology appointments and T1D-related sick days;

f. Alternate arrangements for time missed when blood sugar is out of range; and

g. Full participation in sports, extracurricular activities, and field trips

Naturally, the kinds of accommodations in a 504 plan will depend on the age, maturity, and competence of the particular student. For example, many high school students' 504 plans state that they are allowed to give themselves insulin in school. Most elementary school students' 504 plans state that they are *not* allowed to give themselves insulin in school and that the school nurse or another trained staff member must give them insulin when needed.

7. Accommodations should be used only under legitimate circumstances. Do not abuse your accommodations!

T1D dad tip: Every year, I request all the possible accommodations my T1D child may ever reasonably need. If he needs an accommodation, it's there and he can use it. At the same time, I emphasize to him that he should always be truthful about his Type 1 diabetes and never take unfair advantage of his accommodations.

8. If a student with Type 1 qualifies for special education, he is entitled to special education in addition to a 504 plan for his T1D.

9. At the beginning of every school year, a student's 504 should be reviewed, modified if necessary, and signed by an appropriate school staff member and parent. A 504 plan can be amended at any time during the school year if circumstances change.

10. A student may also be entitled to certain accommodations for standardized tests like the SAT or ACT because of Type 1 diabetes. Deadlines to apply for accommodations are often far in advance of an actual exam date. Ask the school counselor for help applying for accommodations for standardized testing.

11. College students are also protected from discrimination because of Type 1 diabetes, but the rules and procedures which apply in college are in some ways different than they were in kindergarten - 12th grade. Before starting college, a student with T1D should contact the college's Disability Services Office to apply for accommodations during college because of T1D.

12. A school nurse is not expected to be an expert on Type 1 diabetes. Although she may have learned about it in nursing school, she may not have practical experience managing the disease. Many parents meet with the school nurse (or other staff members who will provide T1D care at school) to provide in-person instruction.

13. Parents should give the school nurse a complete set of all the diabetes supplies their child may need at school, including a lancing device, lancets, a meter, test strips, insulin pens or vials and syringes, an extra infusion set (if on a pump), juice boxes or glucose tablets to treat lows, chargers and extra batteries, if needed, and a glucagon kit. Place all of the supplies (other than unopened insulin, which the nurse can keep refrigerated in her office) in a container labeled with the student's name.

14. Parents should also give the school nurse the parents' contact information and the child's endocrinologist's contact information in case of emergency.

15. Work with the school nurse to replenish diabetes supplies which have been used or which have expired.

16. Be polite and patient with your child's school nurse. Almost always, her intentions are good. If there is an issue, try to resolve it with her promptly and amicably.

T1D mom tip: A good school nurse is worth her weight in gold. Make sure to thank her and acknowledge the work she does for your child at least once every school year. Also, let her supervisor know what a good job she is doing for your child.

<u>*T1D grandmother tip*</u>*: I am raising my grandson, who has Type 1. His school nurse is an angel, and while I'd like to buy her a nice gift, I can't afford to spend much money. To express my gratitude, at the end of every semester, I give her a small bag of individually wrapped candies (total cost is less than one dollar) and a handwritten note thanking her for all the work she does to keep my grandson safe at school.*

<u>*T1D mom tip*</u>*: You want to have the school nurse "in your child's corner." Don't get off on the wrong foot with her. Of course, if a school nurse is negligent or endangers your child, you need to address the situation and take appropriate action, but stick to the facts and avoid disrespectful behavior.*

<u>Summary</u>

- In virtually all schools and colleges, students with T1D are protected from discrimination because of the disease.
- A 504 plan is a written document which acknowledges that a student has T1D and is entitled to certain accommodations at school.
- Having T1D alone gives a student the right to have a 504 plan.

Chapter 24

T1D in the Workplace

> *Every time my know-it-all co-worker talks about diabetes without specifying which type, I passive-aggressively correct her under my breath.*

1. The same laws which protect students with Type 1 diabetes from discrimination in school (Section 504 and the Americans with Disabilities Act) **also protect employees with Type 1 diabetes from discrimination in the workplace.**

2. Type 1 diabetes is considered to be a *disability* under these laws. Sometimes, PWD object to the word *disability* because they don't think of Type 1 as a disability. The meaning of "disability" under these particular laws, however, is different from the meaning of "disability" in ordinary language. Because Type 1 diabetes is considered to be a disability *under these particular laws*, employees with Type 1 are entitled to certain legal protections.

3. Generally, a PWD is not legally required to tell a prospective employer that she has diabetes before she is offered a job. Once she has accepted a job offer, though, if she wants to request accommodations, she must tell her employer about her diabetes.

4. Apart from having Type 1 diabetes, an employee must be qualified for the job in question. A qualified worker is one who has the skill, experience, education, and other job-related requirements for the position, and who -- if given reasonable accommodations -- can perform the essential functions of the position.

5. The laws protecting people with T1D in the workplace provide that employers with 15 or more employees:

    a. Cannot ask about an applicant's health status before making a job offer;

    b. Cannot fail to hire, fail to promote, or fire a person with T1D because of her diabetes, unless there is a significant risk of substantial harm which cannot be eliminated with accommodations;

    c. Must not discriminate against people with T1D with regard to employer-provided health insurance; and

    d. Must make reasonable accommodations for a PWD who asks for them to help her perform the essential functions of her job, unless doing so would cause an undue hardship on the employer because of significant difficulty or expense

6. Fortunately, the accommodations which people with Type 1 diabetes need are usually easy and inexpensive. One example is allowing a PWD to take a break from work to check her blood sugar and treat it if necessary.

7. In the United States, a person with Type 1 can become a law enforcement officer, firefighter, or commercial driver as long as she meets certain standards which each of those professions requires to ensure her and the public's safety. `

8. There are very few jobs which people are not allowed to do because they have Type 1 diabetes. In the United States, however, a person with Type 1 cannot enlist in the uniformed services of the military.

<u>Summary</u>

- A person with Type 1 diabetes is not legally required to tell a prospective employer that she has T1D.
- Generally, employers are required to grant reasonable accommodations to employees because of their T1D.
- Generally, employers cannot fire a person with T1D because of her diabetes.

Chapter 25

Traveling with T1D

Murphy's Law of Type 1 diabetes: If something can go wrong when you're traveling with T1D, it will.

The secret to smooth travel with T1D is preparing in advance for anything and everything to go wrong.

1. Every day, people who have Type 1 diabetes travel domestically and internationally. The key to successful travel with T1D is preparation. Plan in advance not only to be able to manage diabetes while traveling, but also for the possibility of something going wrong, like a flight being delayed, canceled, or diverted.

2. When choosing destinations, think about what you will do during your trip if you have a Type 1 diabetes health emergency or a non-T1D health situation/ emergency, which may also affect your diabetes.

3. Bring all of your diabetes supplies with you and keep them close at hand when you travel. To be safe, bring double the number of supplies you expect to use while you are away. This is so that you are prepared in case you have a malfunction or other mishap, or in case of theft, damage, or loss.

4. In addition to all your usual diabetes supplies, remember to pack a glucagon kit, chargers (and electrical adapters, if necessary), extra batteries (if applicable), snack food, water, and backup supplies (e.g., backup insulin pens and needles if your insulin pump stops working). Some insulin pump companies will let you borrow a "loaner" pump while traveling to use if your own pump fails.

5. When traveling internationally, it is helpful to bring paper prescriptions for all your diabetes supplies in case you need to fill a prescription during your time abroad. Some pharmacies in other countries will only accept paper prescriptions.

6. Always wear your medical ID bracelet or other medical identification when you travel.

7. When you fly, never check any bag containing diabetes supplies. Checked baggage or its contents can be lost, stolen, or damaged. Contents can also be subject to extreme heat or cold, which can ruin insulin and other supplies. **Instead, pack your diabetes supplies in a carry-on bag which will fit in the overhead compartment or under the seat in front of you.** If a flight attendant wants you to gate-check the bag, explain that you can't because you have Type 1 diabetes and your bag contains medical supplies which you must have near you at all times. Make sure your supplies and your bag are labeled with your name and telephone number in case of loss.

8. When going through a security checkpoint at an airport, inform security agents that you have Type 1 diabetes and are carrying necessary medical supplies. While not absolutely necessary, it can be helpful to have a doctor's note with you stating that you have T1D and need to have your medication and other supplies (including juice boxes and/ or water) with you at all times. Pack supplies in their own clear, sealable bags so they can be identified easily. **The general rule prohibiting passengers from carrying more than three ounces of liquids or gels through a security checkpoint does not apply to insulin, glucagon, or other liquids and gels used in diabetes management.**

9. If you are wearing a pump or CGM, inform security personnel when you are at the head of the line. A pump or CGM can go through a metal detector, but they should never go through an X-ray machine or body scanner. Unless you choose to remove your pump and CGM, you should request a pat-down and visual inspection because of your medical devices.

10. Unlike today's smart phones, the time on diabetes devices doesn't automatically change when you enter a new time zone. Remember to manually change the time on your devices when you enter a new time zone. (Whether you're traveling or not, change the time on your devices as necessary at the beginning and end of Daylight Saving Time.)

11. No matter what form of transportation you use to travel, pay attention to temperature. Insulin which becomes too hot or too cold will no longer be effective. Some people use cold packs when they travel. (Be careful using ice packs because you don't want your insulin to freeze.) Many people with Type 1 use insulin cooling cases which are specifically designed to keep insulin pens and vials in the recommended temperature range.

12. Most hotels will grant a request to have a small refrigerator, if available, in your hotel room to keep insulin refrigerated during your stay.

<u>T1D mom tip</u>: Before my college son left the United States to study abroad, I worked with his endocrinologist, pharmacist, and insurance company to get a "vacation override." As a result, before he left the U.S., he had all the supplies he would need for the entire time he would be abroad, and our insurance company covered its share of the cost.

<u>T1D mom confession</u>: If someone had told me at the time of my 16-year-old daughter's diagnosis that four years later, she would fly by herself to the other side of the world to study abroad for a semester, I never would have believed it.

<u>T1D young adult tip</u>: I ran out of insulin when I was studying abroad in Paris. I went to a local pharmacy to get a vial, and was surprised when the pharmacist said she couldn't fill the prescription without a paper "script." Fortunately, I knew another PWD in my program who was able to lend me a vial. From then on, I've always brought hard copies of my prescriptions with me when I travel abroad.

<u>T1D adult tip</u>: Whenever I travel, I bring snacks which don't have to be refrigerated. My current favorites are peanut butter crackers and protein bars.

<u>T1D mom tip</u>: I don't feel comfortable having my teenager travel to locations where he can't get prompt, high-quality medical care in case of emergency. Last year, I told him that he couldn't go on a week-long mission trip to a remote location which had been ravaged by a hurricane. He was disappointed, but in the end, he understood my concern. Instead, he was able to volunteer on a week-long service project a few hours from our home.

<u>Summary</u>

With advance planning and extra diabetes prescription and non-prescription supplies, people with T1D are able to travel successfully domestically and internationally.

Chapter 26

The Artificial Pancreas

1. The artificial pancreas (AP) is a technology to treat Type 1 diabetes which researchers have been working on and improving for years. It is NOT a cure.

2. Contrary to the image the name suggests, the artificial pancreas is NOT a man-made organ implanted in the body.

3. The AP is medical equipment which attaches to the outside of a patient's body. It is intended to mimic the function of a healthy pancreas, i.e., to work as a "closed loop" system. Researchers haven't yet developed an artificial pancreas which works as perfectly as a healthy, natural pancreas. With that goal in mind, though, they continue to improve and refine the AP.

4. The artificial pancreas consists of an insulin pump and a continuous glucose monitor (CGM) which work together as a system. Both are attached to the patient's body. The pump and the CGM communicate wirelessly with each other. A sophisticated *algorithm* (a step-by-step computer formula) evaluates the data provided by the CGM to adjust the pump's insulin delivery. **The goal is to keep the user's blood sugar in the target range as much as possible without severe hypoglycemic or hyperglycemic events.**

5. The AP is being made available to patients in stages. Currently, there are several hybrid artificial pancreas systems used by people with T1D.

The early 2020 versions of the AP are considered to be better than other devices in that they automatically do *some* of the work of diabetes management for the patient, and keep the patient's BG in the target range more of the time than other devices were able to do.

You can expect insulin pump companies to release increasingly sophisticated AP systems in the coming years.

6. Researchers are also working on a "dual hormone" artificial pancreas, which will contain the hormones insulin *and* glucagon. At this time, the hybrid APs on the market only contain insulin.

7. It is estimated that thousands of people worldwide currently use do-it-yourself (DIY) artificial pancreas systems. DIY systems combine FDA-approved insulin pumps and continuous glucose monitors with non-FDA-approved open source software to deliver continuous doses of insulin to the user. OPENAPS, Loop, and Android APS are the most popular of these DIY artificial pancreas systems. In general, people who use DIY systems have reported benefits including more time in range, less hypoglycemia, and better nighttime sleep because of fewer overnight high and low blood sugars. One person known to be using a DIY system had an adverse result which required medical intervention from too much insulin being given. Because the DIY systems haven't gone through the clinical trials and scientific scrutiny required for FDA approval, they don't have the assurance of safety which most patients and health care providers demand.

Summary

- The artificial pancreas is a technology to treat (not cure) T1D, consisting of an insulin pump and a CGM which communicate wirelessly.
- An artificial pancreas automatically does *some* of the work of diabetes management for the user, reducing the burden of diabetes management and the risk of complications associated with Type 1 diabetes.

Chapter 27

Newer to Market Insulins, CGMs, and Glucagons

*All I want for my birthday this year
is for my insurance company to cover
the new CGM my endo prescribed for me.*

1. *Afrezza* is an inhalable insulin which is breathed in through the lungs, not injected or infused. It is approved only for non-smoking adults; it is not known if it is safe for children to use. Afrezza is not a substitute for long-acting insulin, so PWD who use Afrezza must still inject or infuse their long-acting basal insulin.

2. *Fiasp* is an injectable ultra-rapid-acting insulin which starts to work sooner after injection than rapid-acting insulins. It is approved for adults and children two years and older. Fiasp users also must still inject or infuse their long-acting basal insulin.

3. The **Dexcom G6** and the **FreeStyle Libre** are continuous glucose monitors which are, generally, considered accurate enough to use to make insulin dosing decisions without finger-sticks.

4. The *Eversense* is a CGM with a sensor which is implanted by a physician and can be worn for up to 90 days.

5. The *InPen* is a smart insulin pen with some features which until recently were unique to insulin pumps. The smart pen works wirelessly to record mealtime injection data, keep track of insulin on board (the amount of active insulin in a person's body), and calculate bolus insulin.

6. The ***Xeris*** glucagon rescue pen is a liquid glucagon pen for the treatment of severe hypoglycemia.

7. ***Baqsimi*** nasal glucagon is a device which delivers glucagon as a dry powder spray for the treatment of severe hypoglycemia.

<u>Summary</u>

Type 1 diabetes management is continually advancing with new insulins, CGMs, and glucagons, offering people with T1D more choices, better control, and less burdensome diabetes management.

Chapter 28

Other Promising Research

*The ideal is to have a cure for T1D,
but I'd also be thrilled with a new treatment
which would automatically manage
my daughter's diabetes for her
with very little effort on her part.*

1.   There is a lot of promising Type 1 diabetes research being done, focusing on better treatments, prevention, treating and reversing complications, and, of course, finding a cure for T1D. Noteworthy current research projects include:

    a.   *The Artificial Pancreas* (see Chapter 26) - increasingly sophisticated artificial pancreas systems which will automate blood sugar management for people living with Type 1, greatly reducing the health risks associated with T1D and the burden of diabetes management;

    One outstanding example is the "iLet Bionic Pancreas," developed by T1D dad Dr. Ed Damiano and his team. Although it is not yet commercially available, the iLet has been successful in clinical trials. Unlike other hybrid AP systems, the iLet doesn't require users to count carbohydrates and enter carb quantities into their pumps.

    b.   *Smart Insulin* (aka Glucose-Responsive Insulin) - a single dose of insulin that circulates in the bloodstream and turns on when it's needed and off when it's not;

c. *Beta Cell Regeneration* - treatments which restore the body's ability to create healthy beta cells (which produce insulin);

d. *Stem Cells* - transforming stem cells into insulin-producing beta cells;

e. *Beta Cell Replacement* - implanting healthy, insulin-producing beta cells back into the bodies of people with Type 1 diabetes; and

f. *Immunotherapy* - therapies aimed at stopping the immune system attack that causes Type 1 diabetes

2. There is a lot to learn when you are diagnosed with T1D. The science and research continue to advance, so it is important to continue to learn. Patients and caregivers should feel hopeful that current and future research will further reduce the burden of diabetes management and improve both short and long-term health.

<u>Summary</u>

There is a lot of sophisticated and promising research being done to prevent, treat, reverse, and cure Type 1 diabetes and its complications.

Chapter 29

JDRF and other Diabetes-Related Organizations

I finally found my people!

No one else "gets it" like another T1D parent.

1. *JDRF* (originally named the Juvenile Diabetes Research Foundation) **is the leading non-profit organization funding Type 1 diabetes medical research with the goals of preventing, treating, and curing T1D.** Since its creation, JDRF has funded more than $2.2 billion in research.

JDRF chapters do outreach to newly-diagnosed patients with T1D, run fundraising events, and hold programming to educate and provide support to patients and their families.

JDRF also does advocacy work, including running JDRF Children's Congress, a program in which children with Type 1 advocate for government funding of T1D research.

2. The ***American Diabetes Association (ADA)*** is a non-profit organization which also funds medical research, does advocacy work, runs fundraising events, and provides education and support, but -- unlike JDRF -- it is not dedicated exclusively to people with Type 1 diabetes. The ADA is for the benefit of those with *all* types of diabetes and pre-diabetes. **The ADA also runs summer *diabetes camps* for children with T1D.**

88

3. Beyond Type 1 is a non-profit organization focusing on education, advocacy and the path to a cure for Type 1. It also includes programs for those with T2D. Beyond Type 1 collaborates with JDRF to maximize both organizations' efforts to fund T1D medical research.

4. T1International is a non-profit charity which gives local communities the tools to advocate for PWD to have access to affordable insulin and diabetes supplies.

*T1D mom tip: My 11-year-old son was reluctant to go to diabetes camp, but I insisted that he try it. He ended up loving camp and improving his diabetes management skills. Most importantly, he connected and bonded with other campers (his **diabuddies**), who understand what it's like to live with T1D in a way that his non-T1D friends simply can't.*

Summary

- JDRF is the leading non-profit organization funding medical research for T1D.
- The American Diabetes Association does work on behalf of people with all types of diabetes, not just Type 1. The ADA also runs diabetes camps for children with diabetes.

Chapter 30

Famous People with Type 1 Diabetes; People with T1D in Health Care

> *When you see someone else with a CGM or insulin pump and you think, "One of us, he's one of us!"*

1. **Many famous people have T1D.** They include:

    - United States Supreme Court Justice Sonia Sotomayor;
    - British Prime Minister Theresa May;
    - Author Anne Rice;
    - Actors Mary Tyler Moore, Jean Smart, Victor Garber, Elizabeth Perkins, Vanessa Williams, Brec Bassinger, and Mary Mouser;
    - Musicians Nick Jonas, Bret Michaels, Crystal Bowersox, Sheku Kanneh-Mason (who played at the 2018 wedding of Prince Harry and Meghan Markle), and Este Haim;
    - Miss America pageant winner Nicole Johnson;
    - Model Lila Moss (daughter of supermodel Kate Moss), who often shows her pump and CGM on the runway and red carpet;
    - Miss Idaho pageant winner Sierra Sandison (who wore her insulin pump clipped to her bikini during the swimsuit competition);
    - Professional football players Jay Cutler, Kendall Simmons, and Mark Andrews;
    - Professional baseball players Sam Fuld, Adam Duvall, and Brandon Morrow;
    - Professional basketball player Lauren Cox;
    - Professional golfer Kelly Kuehne;

- Professional ice hockey players Bobby Clarke, Nick Boynton, and Max Domi;
- Professional soccer players Scott Allan, Antonia Goransson and Borja Mayoral;
- Professional softball player Sara Groenewegen;
- Olympic cross-country skier Kris Freeman;
- Olympic field hockey athlete Carsten Fischer;
- Olympic swimmer Gary Hall, Jr.
- Professional race car drivers Conor Daly, Dexter Bean, and Charlie Kimball; and
- Entrepreneur and record company executive Damon Dash

2. Others with T1D who have impressed the T1D community in the last few years include:

- Eric Tozer, who in 2019, ran seven marathons on seven continents in seven days; and
- Evelyn Riddell, who in 2018, modeled for an Aerie ad campaign showing her insulin pump and CGM

3. Many people with T1D have gone on to careers in endocrinology and other areas of health care. Some (including current JDRF President and CEO Aaron Kowalski, PhD) have dedicated their professional careers to T1D advocacy and research. It is inspiring to come across endocrinologists, certified diabetes educators, nurses, dietitians, mental health professionals, research scientists, and professional advocates who have T1D themselves.

Summary

People with T1D continue to prove that they are capable of extraordinary intellectual, creative, and physical achievements.

Chapter 31

Rising Cost of Insulin;
T1D as a Pre-Existing Condition

> *"Let's go to Canada for our vacation and we can stock up on insulin. Even with the cost of airfare, hotels, and meals, we will still come out ahead."*

1. T1D can be a very expensive disease to manage. Good health insurance is invaluable for T1D patients and their families. If a PWD is uninsured, underinsured, or has health insurance but can't afford to pay the policy's premiums, deductibles or co-pays, he must look into other options. He may be eligible for government insurance programs like Medicaid/ Medical Assistance or CHIP. He may also be eligible for special programs or coupons offered by pharmaceutical companies. If you need financial help, start by asking a member of the diabetes team in your endocrinologist's office. The ***Diabetes Online Community (DOC)*** is also a good resource for information about affording T1D supplies and treatment.

2. In the United States, between 2002 and 2013, the average list price of insulin nearly tripled.

3. A 2018 study showed that 25% of people with diabetes have rationed or discontinued insulin because of cost. Several people have even died as a result.

4. Many in the T1D community are working to: (a) bring public awareness to this issue; (b) pressure the pharmaceutical companies which make insulin to lower and/ or cap their prices; and (c) get state and federal laws passed to lower or cap insulin prices. By April of

2020, five states (Colorado, Illinois, Minnesota, New Mexico, and Virginia) had passed laws making insulin more affordable under certain circumstances.

5. So-called "Wal-Mart insulin," a cheap version of insulin sold at Wal-Mart under the brand name ReliOn, is an old version of insulin. It does not work as well as the insulin formulations which are currently recommended to treat Type 1 diabetes.

6. The Affordable Care Act (ACA, aka "Obamacare") prohibits insurance companies from discriminating against people with pre-existing conditions. Type 1 diabetes is a pre-existing condition.

7. In many countries, patients pay significantly less for insulin than patients do in the United States. Americans pay more than ten times as much for insulin as Canadians do, according to a commentary published in the New England Journal of Medicine.

Summary

- Type 1 diabetes is an expensive disease to manage. Many Americans are uninsured, underinsured, or can't afford to pay their premiums, deductibles, or co-pays.
- The list price of insulin has nearly tripled in the past decade.
- People in the T1D community are working to make insulin affordable for everyone who needs it.

Chapter 32

Coping with Type 1 Diabetes

> *Diabetes is a full-time job. Except you don't get paid, you never get vacation time, and you can't quit.*
>
> *"Happy Diaversary to my Diabuddy!"*
> *Wait, "happy" isn't the right word.*
> *"Congratulations"? No, that isn't right either.*
>
> *Life doesn't have to be perfect to be beautiful.*

1. For many parents and patients, getting a Type 1 diabetes diagnosis feels like being hit by a truck. Then, as soon as the diagnosis is made, you must learn in two or three days how to manage T1D to keep your loved one or yourself alive. For most people, this is overwhelming.

2. If this was your reaction, know that you are not alone. Impossible as it seems to believe, many others have gotten through this and you can too.

3. Your life has just changed dramatically. Acknowledge this and give yourself permission to grieve the loss of your old life without Type 1 diabetes. Many people observe that dealing with a T1D diagnosis is like going through the "stages of grief" which people go through when dealing with death: denial, anger, bargaining, depression, and acceptance.

4. Try, though, not to get stuck in the grief process. (Easier said than done, I know.) Don't continue to beat yourself up because you missed the signs of Type 1 diabetes; doing so doesn't do anyone any good. If you continue to feel sad or anxious and these feelings are having a negative impact on you or your family, seek support and/ or professional help.

5. Diabetes management is a lot of work -- 24 hours a day, 7 days a week, 365 days a year. You never get a day -- or even half a day -- off. Most PWD regularly have some high and low blood sugar levels which make them feel unwell. Diabetes symptoms and management interrupt patients' and caregivers' sleep. Fear and worry often lurk in the background. **It's completely understandable, then, that Type 1 diabetes may have a negative effect on the mental health of patients and caregivers.**

6. Diabetes affects the entire family, not just the person who has it. Often, parents find themselves arguing more than usual after their child is diagnosed with T1D. Siblings of the child may be afraid that they're also going to get it, or they may be jealous of special attention which their brother or sister who has T1D is getting. Children with Type 1 may feel angry that they were diagnosed with the disease while their siblings were not. Some patients feel self-conscious or embarrassed about their diabetes when they are with their peers or out in public.

    Recognize that Type 1 diabetes is a stressor which can affect feelings and relationships. Feeling sad, guilty, irritable, resentful, or angry makes living with T1D and managing it even harder. If you or someone you care about is struggling, ask for support or professional help. Seeking professional help is a sign of strength, not weakness. **If a patient or caregiver's mental health is not good, diabetes management may suffer. Don't delay seeking help because you assume that nothing can be done. Mental health conditions are treatable. Many PWD and their caregivers have found counseling and/ or medication to be enormously helpful for them in coping with Type 1 diabetes.**

7. Although they usually mean well, friends and relatives may not be able to offer you the level of understanding, comfort, and support which you can get from other PWD or their caregivers. Join an in-person or online support group. Contact your local JDRF chapter and request a Type 1 diabetes mentor. Connect with others in the T1D community. **Having support is critical to successful diabetes management.**

8. Educate yourself. Learn about T1D from your diabetes team and other reliable sources. Talk to other parents and patients. Knowledge is empowering and, in time, your competence and confidence will increase.

T1D treatments, technologies, and research continue to evolve and advance, so your education must be ongoing.
Don't assume that a layperson -- even a layperson with T1D or her caregiver -- always knows what she's talking about. People on the Internet and elsewhere often claim to have expertise, but may provide incorrect information or advice which runs the gamut from unfounded to harmful.

9. Don't expect perfection and don't feel pressure to have perfect numbers in diabetes management. Many factors affect blood sugar and Type 1 diabetes can be unpredictable. Even if you always manage T1D exactly as you are supposed to, you will not always get perfect results.

10. As a general rule, try to integrate diabetes management into the life of a PWD instead of integrating her life into diabetes management. A child or adult who has T1D isn't her disease; she's much more than that. (The author of this book intentionally avoided referring to a person with Type 1 diabetes as a "Type 1 diabetic" to be sensitive to some people who feel that the term labels and defines someone by their illness, when they are, of course, much more than just their illness.)
You may hear parents of children with T1D give the advice, "Let kids be kids," or "Kids first, diabetes second." This is good advice as long as it is applied within reason.

11. Do not punish your child with T1D for mistakes in diabetes management. Children, including teenagers, can't be expected to manage their diabetes the way an adult can. Even adults make mistakes in diabetes management; no one is perfect. Punishing your child for mistakes in T1D management will likely demoralize her, have a negative effect on her mental health, and make her more inclined to lie to you about her diabetes management. Your child didn't cause her Type 1 diabetes. She needs your love and support to manage her disease successfully, to run the figurative marathon which Type 1 diabetes feels like. Many children and teens struggle with T1D management, but eventually mature and go on to take good care of themselves. No matter how hard your child's Type 1 diabetes may be on you, it will always be harder on her.

"Do not punish" does not mean "ignore." By all means, if your child is not doing what she can reasonably be expected to do, talk to her about it. Involve your endocrinologist or other members of the diabetes team; they have likely encountered the same problems with other patients and may be able to help you and your child improve your particular situation.

T1D mom tip: I felt traumatized when my five-year-old son was diagnosed in DKA. On his third day in the hospital, a CDE (who was also a T1D mom herself) noticed how frightened and sad I looked. She took me aside and said, "It will get easier -- not easy -- but easier." I really appreciated her words, which were reassuring, but not falsely optimistic. They proved true for me. Now, whenever I learn of another T1D mom or dad whose child is newly diagnosed, I share that same advice.

T1D mom confession: My 17-year-old daughter went to a friend's birthday party and ate the Italian food and birthday cake which were served. She estimated the carbs and injected the corresponding amount of insulin she would need. She came home a few hours later and her blood sugar was over 300 mg/dL. When she told me this, I rolled my eyes, said her name with a disappointed tone, and told her to correct the high.

Later, I told another T1D mom what had happened, and she replied: "All she did was EAT FOOD -- AND she dosed for it! It's not like she was drinking or using illegal drugs!"

Hearing that made me realize that I had been wrong. I went back to my daughter and apologized for the way I had reacted. I told her that I didn't know what it was like to have Type 1, and reaffirmed that I would always be there to support her.

T1D dad confession: I removed my son's CGM when he stayed overnight at my house because the alarm kept waking me up and I couldn't get any sleep. When I told his mom, she pointed out to me that he is a child, that it interferes with his sleep too, and that ultimately it is my responsibility to make sure that he stays safe when he is with me. I realized that she was right and that I had acted in my own best interest -- not in my son's. I apologized to my ex-wife and my son and resolved never to do that again.

<u>T1D mom tip</u>: I've heard of other Type 1 parents who have taken away their children's insulin pumps and made them go back to multiple daily injections as punishment for poor diabetes management. That appalls me.

I can't understand how it does any good to punish your child with more needle sticks for a disease that isn't their fault.

<u>T1D mom confession</u>: While vacuuming, I found candy wrappers hidden under my son's bed. I felt angry and planned to confront him when he got home from school. I posted about the situation online in one of my T1D groups. Many parents commented that they had also come across their kids' hidden candy stashes. They advised me that confronting him was the worst reaction I could have. It would make him more likely to hide food from me in the future and make him hate T1D more than he already did.

Instead, they suggested that I tell him calmly that I found some candy wrappers when I was cleaning and that I don't want him to feel that he has to hide candy or any other food from me. If he wants to eat candy or anything else, he may, but he just needs to get enough insulin to cover the carbs to stay healthy -- and that's what I care about the most. I followed this advice and it was definitely the right way to go.

<u>Summary</u>

- Getting a Type 1 diabetes diagnosis and having to learn quickly how to manage the disease is very stressful. If you are having difficulty adjusting to the fact that you or your loved one has T1D, seek help and support.
- T1D must be managed 24 hours a day, 7 days a week, 365 days a year. Sometimes, PWD or their parents reach a point where they are not doing well, emotionally and/or physically. If that happens, seek help and support.
- Try to fit diabetes management into the life of a PWD instead of fitting the person's life into diabetes management.

Afterword

If you are reading this book, it's likely that you or someone you care for has Type 1 diabetes. Nothing you do can change that reality right now, but everything you do can change the future.

In 2015, thirty days after the sudden, unexpected death of her husband Dave, businesswoman Sheryl Sandberg wrote a post on Facebook which quickly went viral:

*"I was talking to ... [a friend] about a father-child activity that Dave is not here to do. We came up with a plan to fill in for Dave. I cried to him, "But I want Dave. I want Option A." He put his arm around me and said, "Option A is not available. So let's just kick the s**t out of option B."*

*"Dave, to honor your memory and raise your children as they deserve to be raised, I promise to do all I can to kick the s**t out of Option B..."*

This post affected me deeply. Jenny had been diagnosed with Type 1 diabetes over a year before Sandberg's post was written, but there continued to be many days when I still found myself wishing for our version of Option A. Reading and re-reading Sandberg's post made me truly understand and accept that our version of Option A was not available. The reality was that we *only* had Option B. And, like Sandberg, I was going to raise Jenny as she deserved to be raised, despite T1D. Together, we were going to kick the s**t out of Option B.

Every year, we have a small celebration for Jenny's **diaversary** (the anniversary of the date on which she was diagnosed with Type 1). Occasionally, another T1D parent will balk at the idea of *celebrating* the date of a child's diagnosis. "Why would I want to celebrate the day we learned that she has a serious chronic illness?" the parent will ask.

My answer to that question is that we don't celebrate the *illness*. We celebrate all the hard work our daughter has done in the past year, and the strength and resilience she has shown in managing her T1D. We recognize that there were some bad days, but most were good. We acknowledge the support she has gotten from family and friends. We feel grateful for insulin, her pump, her CGM, and the team of medical professionals who treat her. We know that T1D treatment will continue to improve, and that she will benefit from these advances. We celebrate her life and feel hopeful about her future.

Glossary

(Including common abbreviations, acronyms, and slang)

I am fluent in two languages --
English and Type 1 diabetes.

A

A1c (aka HbA1c or Hemoglobin A1c) - a blood test which measures a person's average overall blood glucose level for the previous 2 - 3 months

Accommodations - special rules/ modifications of general rules applicable to a student in school, or to an employee in the workplace, because of her Type 1 diabetes

Afrezza - an inhalable insulin which is breathed in through the lungs, not injected or infused, approved for use in adults under certain conditions

Algorithm - a step-by-step computer formula

American Diabetes Association (ADA) - a non-profit organization for the benefit of those with all types of diabetes. The ADA also runs diabetes camps for children with diabetes.

Americans with Disabilities Act (ADA) - a federal law prohibiting discrimination against people with Type 1 diabetes (and others) in school and in the workplace

Artificial Pancreas (AP) - a technology consisting of an insulin pump and continuous glucose monitor, which work together to automate insulin delivery

Autoimmune disease - a disease in which the body's own immune system mistakenly attacks part of the body

B

Basal Insulin (aka "background insulin" or "circulating insulin") - insulin given by injection or insulin pump which helps keep blood sugar steady overnight and between meals

Baqsimi glucagon - nasal glucagon delivered as a dry powder spray for the treatment of severe hypoglycemia

Beta Cells - the cells in the pancreas which make insulin

BG - see Blood Glucose

Blood Glucose (BG; aka "blood sugar") - glucose in the blood; also used to mean the amount or level of glucose in the blood

Blood Glucose Level (BGL) - the amount or level of glucose in the blood

Blood Sugar - see Blood Glucose

Bolus Insulin - insulin given by injection or insulin pump to lower increases in BG from meals and snacks, and, if needed, to correct high blood sugar

C

Cannula - a tiny, flexible tube inserted under the skin, through which insulin is delivered

Carbohydrate (carb) - the nutrient in food which raises blood sugar more than any other nutrient

Certified Diabetes Educator (CDE) - a medical professional with advanced training and certification in diabetes management

CGM - see Continuous Glucose Monitor

Chronic - lifelong; doesn't "go away"

Closed Loop System - in a person without T1D, the system in which the pancreas automatically produces the correct amount of insulin needed to move blood sugar from the bloodstream into the cells

Complications - the long-term health problems which people with T1D may develop as a result of years of poorly-controlled blood sugar

Continuous Glucose Monitor (CGM) - a very small device attached to the body which measures the user's blood sugar level

Correction Bolus or Correction Dose - bolus insulin given to lower blood sugar to one's target BG

Count/ Counting Carbohydrates (aka counting carbs) - determining how many grams of carbohydrate are in a particular snack or meal

Cover/ Covering Carbohydrates (aka covering carbs) - giving an amount of insulin based on the amount of carbohydrate consumed

D

D - (slang) shorthand for "diabetes"; also used together with other words: D-mom (mom of a child with T1D); D-bag (see Diabetes Bag)

Dexcom G6 - a brand and model of continuous glucose monitor (CGM)

Diabetes Alert Dog (DAD) - a service dog which has been specially trained to sense/ smell a PWD's low blood sugar and alert him and others to it

Diabetes Bag - bag or kit used to carry diabetes supplies

Diabetes Control and Complications Trial (DCCT) - a landmark medical study which proved that intensive management of T1D dramatically reduced the risk of complications from T1D; the DCCT changed the way Type 1 diabetes was treated

Diabetes Online Community (DOC) - the organizations and people who communicate about T1D online

Diabetic Ketoacidosis (DKA) - a serious, life-threatening condition in which ketones build up in the blood as a result of very high blood sugar levels

Diabuddy - a friend who also has T1D

Diaversary - the anniversary of the date of a T1D diagnosis

Dietitian - healthcare professional who teaches PWD about nutrition, how to count carbs, how to match insulin to food consumed, and how to maintain, lose, or gain weight, if needed

DKA - see Diabetic Ketoacidosis

DOC - see Diabetes Online Community

E

Endocrinologist (endo) - a physician who specializes in treating Type 1 diabetes

Eversense CGM - a brand and model of CGM which is implanted by a physician and can be worn for up to 90 days.

F

Family and Medical Leave Act (FMLA) - a federal law which allows employees to take up to 12 weeks of unpaid leave from work to care for a child, spouse, or parent with T1D

<u>Fiasp</u> - an injectable ultra-rapid-acting insulin which starts to work sooner after injection than rapid-acting insulins. It is approved for adults and children two years and older under certain conditions.

<u>Freestyle Libre</u> - a brand and model of continuous glucose monitor (CGM)

<u>G</u>

<u>Glucometer</u> - (see Meter) - a device which measures blood sugar levels

<u>Glucagon</u> - a hormone used to raise blood glucose in a person with severe hypoglycemia

<u>Glucose</u> - the type of sugar which results from the digestive system breaking down food, and which then enters the bloodstream

<u>Gram</u> - a unit of weight in the metric system, often used to measure the amount of carbohydrate in food and drink

<u>H</u>

<u>HbA1c</u> - see A1c

<u>Honeymoon Phase</u> - the limited period of time, beginning after a T1D diagnosis and after insulin has been injected, during which a PWD's pancreas will produce some insulin again

<u>Hyperglycemia</u> - high blood sugar; having too much glucose (sugar) in the blood

<u>Hypoglycemia</u> - low blood sugar; having too little glucose (sugar) in the blood

<u>Hypoglycemia Unawareness</u> - not being able to sense or feel one's own low blood sugar

Infusion - the delivery of insulin from an insulin pump into the body

Infusion Set - a piece of medical equipment through which insulin is delivered from an insulin pump into the body

Inject/ Injection (aka shot) - to deliver, or the delivery of, insulin from a syringe or insulin pen into the body

InPen - a smart insulin pen with some features which until recently were unique to insulin pumps

Insulin - a hormone which regulates blood sugar levels; people who have Type 1 diabetes don't make their own insulin anymore, so they must inject or infuse man-made insulin.

Insulin Pen - a device containing insulin which, with an attached needle, is used to inject insulin

Insulin Pump (aka pump) - a programmable device which attaches to the outside of the body and delivers insulin just beneath the skin

Insulin to Carbohydrate (Carb) Ratio - a personalized ratio indicating that a PWD needs one unit of insulin for a certain number of grams of carbohydrate consumed

Intensive Management (aka Intensive Treatment) - a type of diabetes management which requires frequent blood sugar testing, frequent insulin injections or infusions, adjusting insulin doses according to food consumed, and frequent checkups with a diabetes team

Interstitial Blood Sugar - the blood sugar in the interstitial fluid surrounding the cells; a CGM measures interstitial blood sugar

J

JDRF (formerly known as the Juvenile Diabetes Research Foundation) - the leading non-profit organization funding Type 1 diabetes medical research

K

Ketones - poisonous substances which are produced when there is not enough insulin to move glucose into the body's cells to get energy

Ketone Test Strips - test strips which are used to test urine for the presence and size of ketones

L

Lancing Device (aka Lancer); Lancet - a plastic device which holds a sharp lancet (needle), used to do a finger-stick to measure blood sugar; in slang, aka "poker" or "pricker"

M

Management of T1D - the work (testing blood sugar, injecting or infusing insulin, counting carbs in food, determining insulin doses, correcting high blood sugars, treating low blood sugars, etc.) which is done to properly take care of one's T1D

Meter (aka Glucometer) - a device which measures blood sugar levels

MDIs (see Multiple Daily Injections)

Multiple Daily Injections (MDIs) - many injections every day to deliver insulin into the body

P

<u>Pancreas</u> - the organ in the human body which makes insulin

<u>Pen</u> (see Insulin Pen)

<u>Primary Care Provider</u> (PCP) - the health care provider a PWD sees for preventive and routine care; usually a pediatrician, internist, or family medicine doctor

<u>Pump</u> - (noun) see Insulin Pump; (verb) use an insulin pump

<u>Pumper</u> - a person who uses an insulin pump

<u>PWD</u> - person/ people with diabetes

R

<u>Rule of 15</u> - a general rule that to treat a low blood sugar, a PWD should consume 15 grams of a fast-acting carbohydrate (such as fruit juice or glucose tablets), then wait 15 minutes to check that blood sugar has risen back into the target range

S

<u>Section 504 of the Rehabilitation Act of 1973</u> (aka Section 504) - a federal law prohibiting discrimination against people with Type 1 diabetes in school and in the workplace

<u>Sensor</u> - a tiny part of a CGM which a PWD inserts just below the skin to measure her blood sugar

<u>Sharps Box or Container</u> - the box or container used to safely dispose of old lancets, syringes, needles, test strips, infusion sets, and any other diabetes items which are sharp or have bodily fluids on them; once filled to capacity, a sharps box should be locked

108

<u>Site</u> - location, place, or spot on the body where insulin is injected or infused

<u>Stack/ Stacking</u> - give/ giving insulin doses too close together in time, which is dangerous because it may cause a low BG

<u>Subcutaneously</u> - just beneath the skin

<u>SWAG</u> (scientific wild-ass guess) - slang; (noun) an educated guess, or (verb) making an educated guess, about a food's carb content when nutrition information or food measuring tools aren't available

<u>Syringe</u> - a tube-like device used with a needle to inject insulin

T

<u>T1 or T1D</u> - see Type 1 diabetes

<u>T1D adult/ T1D child/ T1D teen</u> - adult/ child/ teen who has T1D

<u>T1D dad/ T1D mom/ T1D parent</u> - dad/ mom/ parent of a child with T1D

<u>T2D</u> - see Type 2 diabetes

<u>Target Blood Glucose</u> (aka Target Blood Sugar) - the desired blood sugar level (specified by one's diabetes team) to which a PWD should correct his blood sugar

<u>Target Range</u> - the desired range of blood sugar levels (specified by one's diabetes team) in which a person with T1D should try to keep his blood sugar

<u>Test Strip</u> - a strip, compatible with and inserted into a meter, on which a PWD places a small drop of blood to measure her BG level

<u>Tight Control</u> - keeping one's blood sugar levels within the target range as much as possible; intensive T1D management leads to tight control

Time in Range (TIR) - the percentage of time a PWD's blood sugar is in his target range

Type 1 diabetes (aka Type 1 or T1D) - an autoimmune disease in which the body stops making insulin

Type 2 diabetes (aka Type 2 or T2D) - a metabolic disease in which the body has become resistant to the insulin it naturally produces

U

Unicorn - (slang) 1. a BG level of 100 mg/dl; 2. (used less often) when the BG levels on two different devices are identical at the same time

X

Xeris glucagon pen - a liquid glucagon rescue pen for the treatment of severe hypoglycemia

Miscellaneous

504 Plan (aka 504 Agreement) - a legal document stating that a student has T1D, and that because of his disease, certain school rules will be modified for him

References & Resources

<u>Print Books</u>

American Diabetes Association. (2011). *Complete Guide to Diabetes: The Ultimate Home Reference from the Diabetes Experts.* Alexandria, VA: American Diabetes Association.

American Diabetes Association. (2016). *Diabetes A to Z: What You Need to Know about Diabetes -- Simply Put.* Alexandria, VA: American Diabetes Association.

Colberg, S., & Edelman, S.V. (2007). *50 Secrets of the Longest Living People with Diabetes.* Da Capo Press, Perseus Books Group.

Edelman, S. & Friends. (2018). *Taking Control of Your Diabetes.*

West Islip, NY: Professional Communications Inc.

Mayo Clinic. (2014). *The Essential Diabetes Book: How to Prevent, Control, and Live Well with Diabetes.* New York, NY: Time Home Entertainment Inc.

McCarthy, M. (2013). *Raising Teens with Diabetes: A Survival Guide for Parents.* Ann Arbor, MI: Spry Publishing.

Milchovich, S.K., & Dunn-Long, B. (2015). *Diabetes Mellitus: A Practical Handbook.* Boulder, CO: Bull Publishing.

Powell, Lisa. (2010). *Type 1 Diabetes for People Who Don't Have It.* San Bernardino, CA: Lulu.com.

Rubin, A. (2015). *Diabetes for Dummies.* Hoboken, NJ: John Wiley & Sons, Inc.

Scheiner, G. (2012). *Think Like a Pancreas: A Practical Guide to Managing Diabetes with Insulin.* Boston, MA: Da Capo Lifelong Books.

Vieira, G. (2014). *Dealing with Diabetes Burnout: How to Recharge and Get Back on Track When You Feel Frustrated and Overwhelmed Living with Diabetes*. New York, NY: Demos Health.

Walsh, J., & Roberts, R. (2013). *Pumping Insulin: Everything you need for success on an Insulin Pump*. San Diego, CA: Torrey Pines Press.

Warshaw, H.S., & Kulkarni, K. (2011). *The Complete Guide to Carb Counting*. Alexandria, VA: American Diabetes Association.

Wood, J., & Peters, A. (2018). *The Type 1 Diabetes Self-Care*

Manual: A Complete Guide to Type 1 Diabetes Across the Lifespan for People with Diabetes, Parents, and Caregivers. Arlington, VA: American Diabetes Association.

Websites

https://www.ajmc.com/journals/evidence-based-diabetes-management/2019/september-2019/gathering-evidence-on-insulin-rationing-answers-and-future-questions

https://www.ajmc.com/newsroom/fda-approves-fiasp-for-children-with-diabetes

https://bantinghousenhsc.wordpress.com/2018/12/14/insulin-patent-sold-for-1/

https://beyondtype1.org/evelyn-riddell-interview/

https://www.biospace.com/article/new-report-shows-price-of-insulin-doubled-from-2012-to-2016/

https://blog.bluecircle.foundation/diabetes-dictionary/

https://care.diabetesjournals.org/content/41/6/1299

https://www.cdc.gov/diabetes/pdfs/data/statistics/national-diabetes-statistics-report.pdf

https://www.cnn.com/2019/05/23/health/colorado-insulin-price-cap-trnd/index.html

https://www.cnn.com/2019/10/31/politics/faa-pilots-diabetes

https://consumer.healthday.com/diabetes-information-10/insulin-news-414/why-are-insulin-prices-still-so-high-for-u-s-patients-751960.html

https://www.diabetes.org/community/camp

https://www.diabetes.org/diabetes/genetics-diabetes

https://www.diabetes.org/newsroom/press-releases/2019/insulin-price-reduction-act

https://www.diabetes.org/resources/know-your-rights/discrimination/employment-discrimination

https://www.diabetes.org/resources/know-your-rights/discrimination/

public-accommodations-and-government-programs/fact-sheet-discrimination-public-places-and-government-programs

https://www.diabetes.org/resources/know-your-rights/drivers-licenses-laws

https://www.diabetes.org/resources/know-your-rights/safe-at-school-state-laws

https://www.diabetes.org/resources/know-your-rights/safe-at-school-state-laws/special-considerations/common-issues

https://www.diabetes.org/resources/know-your-rights/safe-at-school-state-laws/written-care-plans/diabetes-medical-management-plan

https://www.diabetes.org/resources/know-your-rights/section-504-rehabilitation-act-1973

https://www.diabetesselfmanagement.com/managing-diabetes/getting-to-know-you/nine-athletes-type-1-diabetes/

https://www.espn.com/womens-college-basketball/story/id/27959026/
baylor-lauren-cox-using-basketball-spotlight-inspire-sister-other-
diabetics

https://www.goodrx.com/blog/smoking-diabetes-high-blood-sugar-
insulin-resistance-health-risks/

https://www.health.harvard.edu/blog/can-vaping-damage-your-lungs-
what-we-do-and-dont-know-2019090417734

https://healthcostinstitute.org/diabetes-and-insulin/price-of-insulin-
prescription-doubled-between-2012-and-2016

https://www.healthline.com/diabetesmine/why-not-more-affordable-
generic-insulin#11

https://www.healthline.com/diabetesmine/26-famous-people-with-type-
1-diabetes

https://www.hhs.gov/answers/affordable-care-act/can-i-get-coverage-if-i-
have-a-pre-existing-condition/index.html

https://www.informationaboutdiabetes.com/lifestyle/lifestyle/e-
cigarettes-not-a-safer-smoking-option-with-diabetes-two-studies

https://www.jdrf.org/blog/2019/03/13/eric-tozer-world-marathon-
challenge-recap/

https://www.jdrf.org/blog/2019/04/09/jdrf-names-aaron-kowalski-new-
president-and-ceo/

https://www.jdrf.org/blog/2020/02/18/more-people-being-diagnosed-
type-1-diabetes/

https://www.jdrf.org/impact/advocacy

https://www.jdrf.org/impact/advocacy/special-diabetes-program

https://www.jdrf.org/impact/research

https://www.jdrf.org/t1d-resources/about/facts

https://www.jdrf.org/t1d-resources/about/insulin

https://www.jdrf.org/t1d-resources/technology

https://onlineclasses.joslin.org/info/the_advantages_and_disadvantages_
of_an_insulin_pump.html

http://www.ldonline.org/article/6108

https://www.medicaleconomics.com/article/rising-price-insulin

https://news.yale.edu/2018/12/03/one-four-patients-say-theyve-skimped-
insulin-because-high-cost

https://www.newsweek.com/illinois-becomes-second-state-cap-monthly-
insulin-prices-more-states-are-considering-it-1483987

https://parade.com/68356/parade/stars-with-diabetes/#celebrities-with-
diabetes-tom-hanks-slideshow

https://www.pharmacytimes.com/news/new-mexico-becomes-third-
state-to-cap-monthly-insulin-costs

https://thehill.com/policy/healthcare/486419-virginia-lawmakers-pass-
lowest-insulin-price-cap-in-nation-at-50-a-month

https://www.t1everydaymagic.com/celebrities-with-type-1-diabetes/

https://www.usatoday.com/story/tech/2015/06/03/sheryl-sandberg-
facebookdave-goldberg-death-mourning/28407911

https://www.usnews.com/news/health-news/articles/2019-11-07/why-
are-insulin-prices-still-so-high-for-us-patients

https://www.verywellhealth.com/famous-people-with-type-1-diabetes-
3289472

<u>Select Organizations related to T1D and their Websites</u>

American Diabetes Association (ADA), www.diabetes.org
Beyond Type 1, www.beyondtype1.org

Children with Diabetes, www.childrenwithdiabetes.com
Children's Diabetes Foundation/ Barbara Davis Center for Diabetes,
www.childrensdiabetesfoundation.org
College Diabetes Network (CDN), www.collegediabetesnetwork.org
Connected in Motion, www.connectedinmotion.ca
Helmsley Charitable Trust, www.helmsleytrust.org/programs/health-
type- 1-diabetes
JDRF, www.jdrf.org
Joslin Diabetes Center, www.joslin.org
T1International, www.t1international.com

Select Blogs related to T1D

A Sweet Life
Diabetes Daily
Diabetes Mine
DiaTribe
Insulin Nation
T1 Everyday Magic

Select Facebook Groups related to T1D

Diabetes and Diapers
Parents of Type 1 Diabetics
POKED (Parents of Kids Enduring Diabetes)
Proud parents of athletes with Type 1 diabetes
T1D College Transition: Forum for Parents
T1D Mod Squad (Mod = mothers of diabetics, but dads welcome too)
Type 1 Diabetes and Pregnancy

Select Twitter Hashtags related to T1D

#T1D or #t1d, and #type1diabetes

Podcast

The Juicebox Podcast

Acknowledgements

Just as support is critical to successful diabetes management, it was critical to my writing this book. Thank you to my (and Jenny's) supporters:

- Elise Emanuele Wood, RD, CDE, and person with T1D; Nancy W. Glynn, PhD, T1D mom and my T1D mentor; and Linda Seamonson and other friends and family members, for reading my manuscript and providing helpful comments;

- Lisa Powell, author and T1D mom, Moira McCarthy Stanford, author, journalist, speaker and T1D mom; and Ginger Vieira, author and person with T1D, for sharing advice about the publishing process;

- Ingrid Libman, MD, PhD, pediatric endocrinologist, Children's Hospital of Pittsburgh, Pittsburgh, Pennsylvania and Rachna Goyal, MD, adult endocrinologist, MedStar Georgetown, Washington, DC, for giving Jenny outstanding medical care;

- Cindy Baird, School Nurse Extraordinaire, Upper St. Clair, Pennsylvania (I haven't forgotten that I promised to take you out to lunch when the fully-realized artificial pancreas is available)

- Sharon Helden, dear friend who shoveled several inches of snow from my driveway on the February day when Jenny was discharged from the hospital after her T1D diagnosis;

- The Western & Central Pennsylvania chapter of JDRF and the Gala Committee members I work with every year to raise funds for T1D medical research;

- The T1D moms and dads I've met in person and online through the Diabetes Online Community, for teaching and supporting me and allowing me to teach and support others;

- The extended Pearlman and Park families, and the Seamonson-Mayersohn family, who have always been there for my family;

- My son, Robert, who stepped up and took care of business when Jenny was diagnosed -- although it took him a few months to remember that the individually-labeled snack foods in the fridge and pantry were not for him; and finally,

- My husband, Paul, who did more than his share of overnight blood sugar checks. I can't overestimate the value of his love and support in our family's T1D journey.

Index